MW01076057

DUST OFF:
ARMY AEROMEDICAL
EVACUATION
IN VIETNAM

by

Peter Dorland
and
James Nanney

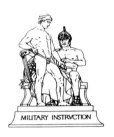

MILITARY INSTRVCTION

CENTER OF MILITARY HISTORY
UNITED STATES ARMY
WASHINGTON, D.C., 2008

Library of Congress Cataloging in Publication Data

Dorland, Peter, 1946–
    Dust Off.

    Bibliography: p.
    Includes index.
    1. Vietnamese Conflict, 1961–1975 — Medical and sanitary affairs. 2.
Vietnamese Conflict, 1961–1975 — Aerial operations, American. I. Nanney,
James, 1945–
II. Center of Military History (U.S.) III. Title.
DS559.44.D67   1982   959.704'37   82–8858
                                                                       AACR2

First Printed 1982—CMH Pub 90–28–1

For sale by the Superintendent of Documents, U.S. Government Printing Office
Internet: bookstore.gpo.gov   Phone: toll free (866) 512-1800;   DC area (202) 512-1800
Fax: (202) 512-2104 Mail: Stop IDCC, Washington, DC 20402-0001

ISBN 978-0-16-075478-4

Foreword

From the wheatfields of the Civil War to the jungles and paddies of Vietman, the United States Army has led the world in adapting modern transport technology to the humanitarian goal of saving the lives of the sick and wounded. Drawing on its first experiments with helicopters in Korea, the Army in Vietnam came to rely almost entirely on the helicopter for medical evacuation. The Dust Off and Medevac helicopter ambulance units tested and perfected for medical use the Army's new helicopter, the UH–1 ("Huey" Iroquois), and developed several new devices, especially the hoist, that helped save thousands of American and allied lives between 1962 and 1973. The pilots of these helicopter ambulances displayed a courage and devotion to duty that earned them widespread respect from soldiers in Vietnam.

This book chronicles the early problems of medical evacuation in Vietnam, recounts the valor of several of the Dust Off crews, and describes the procedures and equipment used to speed the movement of patients to in-theater Army hospitals. It also shows the effect that the helicopter had on traditional Army procedures dating back to the Civil War. It should interest anyone concerned with Army medical history, the Vietnam War, or the problem of administering medical care in war or in times of civilian disasters. The widespread use of the helicopter for medical evacuation in America since the Vietnam War testifies to the broader issues raised by this study, and of the relevance of Army history to the civilian community. It is gratifying that the demand for this work justifies this new reprint.

Washington, D.C.
22 May 1984

DOUGLAS KINNARD
Brigadier General, U.S.A. (Ret.)
Chief of Military History

Preface

During a tour with The Historical Unit, U.S. Army Medical Department, Fort Detrick, Maryland, from 1974 to 1977, Peter G. Dorland, then a captain and a former Dust Off pilot in Vietnam, completed the basic research for this book and drafted a lengthy manuscript. In the first seven months of 1981, as an editor at the U.S. Army Center of Military History (CMH), Washington, D.C., I conducted further research on Dust Off, reorganized and redrafted portions of the original manuscript, and added Chapter 4 and the Epilogue.

The authors accumulated a store of debts, both at Fort Detrick and Washington. Albert E. Cowdrey, chief of the Medical History Branch (CMH), supervised the project, improving the manuscript's prose and organization in many places, and saw that the revision received a review by other historians at the Center: Stanley L. Falk, George L. Mac Garrigle, and Jeffrey Greenhut. Col. James W. Dunn's critical eye also improved the substance of the book. The final editing and preparation of the book for publication was the work of Edith M. Boldan. Arthur S. Hardyman helped design the cover and the map.

Others at the Center who responded to frequent pleas for assistance were Charles Simpson, Col. Mary Van Harn, Charles Ellsworth, Geraldine Judkins, Mary Gillett, Dwight Oland, Graham Cosmas, Vincent Demma, Jeffrey Clarke, and my coworkers in the Editorial Branch.

Without the help of these many people, Peter Dorland and I could not have produced this book. The authors, of course, accept sole responsibility for any errors.

Washington, D.C.   JAMES NANNEY
18 January 1982

The Authors

Peter G. Dorland received a bachelor's degree in biology from Amherst College. From April 1971 to April 1972 he served in Vietnam as an Army lieutenant flying helicopter ambulance missions for "Eagle Dust Off" of the 101st Airborne Division (Airmobile). From 1974 to 1977 he worked on this manuscript at Fort Detrick, Maryland, for the Army Medical Department. He then returned to flying duties, and is currently commanding, as a major, the 247th Medical Detachment at Fort Irwin, California.

James S. Nanney received his B.A., M.A., and Ph.D. degrees from Vanderbilt University. His fields were American diplomatic history and Russian history. From 1974 to 1980 he worked as a research associate for the George C. Marshall Research Foundation, helping Dr. Forrest C. Pogue examine the postwar career of General Marshall as Secretary of State and Secretary of Defense. In 1977–78, he took a year's leave of absence from the Foundation to teach Russian and recent U.S. history at Murray State University, Murray, Kentucky. Since November 1980 he has been a member of the staff of the Center of Military History. He is currently working on the updating of *American Military History*.

Contents

DUST OFF:
ARMY AEROMEDICAL
EVACUATION
IN VIETNAM

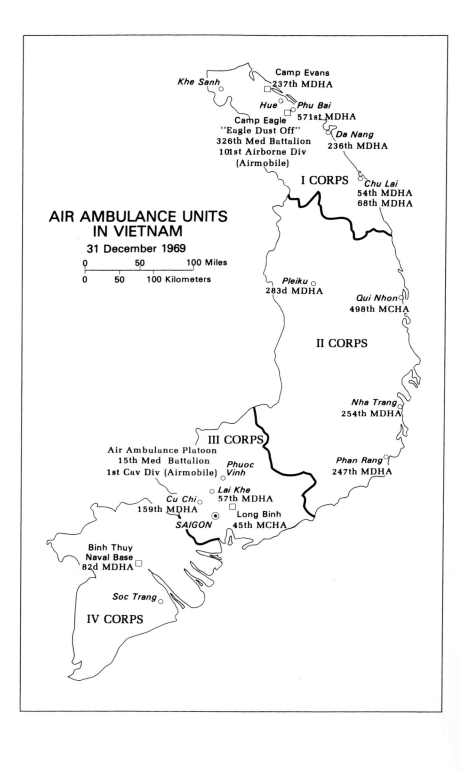

AIR AMBULANCE UNITS
IN VIETNAM

31 December 1969

| 0 | 50 | 100 Miles |
| 0 | 50 | 100 Kilometers |

Khe Sanh

Camp Evans
237th MDHA

Hue Phu Bai
571st MDHA

Camp Eagle
"Eagle Dust Off"
326th Med Battalion
101st Airborne Div
(Airmobile)

Da Nang
236th MDHA

I CORPS

Chu Lai
54th MDHA
68th MDHA

Pleiku
283d MDHA

Qui Nhon
498th MCHA

II CORPS

Nha Trang
254th MDHA

III CORPS

Air Ambulance Platoon
15th Med Battalion
1st Cav Div (Airmobile)

Phuoc
Vinh

Phan Rang
247th MDHA

Cu Chi
159th MDHA

Lai Khe
57th MDHA

Long Binh
45th MCHA

SAIGON

Binh Thuy
Naval Base
82d MDHA

Soc Trang

IV CORPS

CHAPTER I

The Early Years

The small outpost in the Vietnamese delta stood a vigilant watch. For the past twenty-four hours guerrilla soldiers had harassed its defenders with occasional mortar rounds and small arms fire. A radio call for help had brought fighter-bombers and a spotter plane to try to dislodge the enemy from foxholes and bunkers they had built during the night. But neither the aerial observer nor the men in the outpost could detect the Communist soldiers in their concealed positions. At dawn the outpost commander called off his alert and reduced the number of perimeter guards. Then he led a patrol out to survey the area. No sooner had they left their defenses than the enemy opened fire. Two of the soldiers fell, badly wounded, and the rest scrambled back to the safety of their perimeter, dragging their casualties with them.

While the medical corpsmen treated the wounded, a radio telephone operator called their headquarters to the east at Gia Lam. There, when the request for medical evacuation came in, the duty pilot ran to his waiting helicopter and in minutes was airborne. His operations officer had told him that the pickup zone was insecure and that gunships would cover him. Since there were few helicopter ambulances in the theater, this flight would be a long one: forty-five minutes each way. After taking off, the pilots radioed the gunships and confirmed the time and place of rendezvous. On his map he traced his route, out across the paddied landscape, broken only by an occasional village, hamlet, or barbed wire camp.

Five minutes from the beseiged outpost the flight leader of the gunship team radioed the air ambulance that they had him in sight and were closing on him. While the ambulance pilot planned his approach, the gunships made strafing runs over the outpost to keep the enemy down. The outpost commander marked his pickup zone with a smoke grenade, and the ambulance pilot circled down to it from high overhead. As soon as he landed he shouted at the ground troops to load the wounded before a mortar hit him. Once the patients were secured, the pilot sped out of the area and headed toward Lanessan Hospital, radioing ahead to report his estimated time of arrival. Litter bearers from the hospital waited to rush the casualties into the emergency room as soon as the helicopter touched down.

The area where this mission took place was the Red River Delta in northern Vietnam. Gia Lam was the airfield serving Hanoi from across the Doumer Bridge spanning the Red River. The defenders of the outpost were the French in the early 1950s.[1] By the end of 1953 the French in Indochina were using eighteen medical evacuation helicopters. From April 1950 through early 1954 French air ambulances evacuated about five thousand casualties.

In these same years the U.S. Army, which had used a few helicopters for medical evacuation at the end of World War II, employed helicopter ambulances on a larger scale, transporting some 17,700 U.S. casualties of the Korean War. Several years later in the Vietnam War it used helicopter ambulances to move almost 900,000 U.S. and allied sick and wounded. The aeromedical evacuation techniques developed in these wars opened a new era in the treatment of emergency patients. With their ability to land on almost any terrain, helicopters can save precious minutes that often mean the difference between life and death. Today many civilian medical and disaster relief agencies rely on helicopter ambulances. For the past thirty years the U.S. Army has played a leading role in the development of this new technology.

Early Medical Evacuation

Although surgeons often accompanied the professional armies of the eighteenth century, the large citizen armies of the early nineteenth century, whose battles often produced massive casualties, demanded and received the first effective systems of medical evacuation. Two of the officers of Napoleon Bonaparte, the Barons Dominique Jean Larrey and Pierre Francois Percy, designed light, well-sprung carriages for swift evacuation of the wounded. Napoleon saw that each of his divisions received an ambulance corps of about 170 men, headed by a chief surgeon and equipped with the new horse-drawn carriages. Other continental powers quickly adapted the French system to their own needs, but the British and American armies lagged a full half century in learning the medical lessons of the Napoleonic era.

In the Seminole War of 1835–42 in Florida, the U.S. Army Medical Department experimented with horse-drawn ambulances and recommended their adoption by the Army. But the Department apparently got no response. A few years later experiments were resumed, and a four-wheeled ambulance proved successful in the West. But by the outbreak of the Civil War in April 1861 the Army had ac-

---

[1]This incident is related by Valerie André, a French Air Force medical pilot who flew in Indochina, in her article "L'Hélicoptère sanitaire en Indochine," *L'Officier de Réserve*, vol. 2 (1954), pp. 30–31.

quired more two-wheeled than four-wheeled ambulances, and even these were in short supply. In 1862 and 1863 scarce ambulances, poorly trained stretcher bearers, and unruly ambulance drivers greatly hindered the Medical Department's efforts to care for the wounded. Ambulances were so scarce that after the first major battle of the war at Bull Run (21 July 1861) many of the 1,000 Union wounded depended on friends and relatives to pick them up in a family carriage. Many more simply straggled the twenty-five miles back to Washington on foot. Three days after the battle hundreds of wounded still lay where they had fallen. The stretcher bearers consisted almost entirely of members of military bands who had been assigned the duty. As one historian noted, "...scrubbing blood-soaked floors and tables, disposing of dirty scabby bandages and carrying bleeding, shell-shocked soldiers had nothing to do with music, accordingly the impressed musicians fled the scene."

At the second battle of Bull Run (29 August 1862) the large number of civilian drifters hired by the Quartermaster Corps to drive the ambulances simply fled the scene at the first few shots. The Surgeon General quickly rounded up about two hundred more vehicles from the streets of Washington and accepted civilian volunteer drivers, who proved to be worse than the first lot. Many broke into the medicine cabinets on the ambulances, drank the liquor supply, then disappeared. Those who made their way to Bull Run were found stealing blankets and other provisions, and some even took to rifling the pockets of the dead and dying.

Over the course of the war, however, the Union system markedly improved, thanks to the efforts of Maj. Jonathan Letterman, Medical Director of the Army of the Potomac. Letterman recommended sweeping reforms in the ambulance system and the creation of an orderly group of medical clearing stations to the immediate rear of each battlefront. The mission of the ambulances was to bring all casualties to the clearing stations as rapidly as possible. The station would then sort the casualties, a process known as triage. As soon as possible the surgeons went to work on the serious casualties whom they deemed savable and sent them to hospitals in the rear. The most seriously wounded were often set aside, many to die before they reached the operating table. The lightly wounded were treated later and retained near the front. Two goals suffused Letterman's new system: to reduce the time between wounding and lifesaving (definitive) surgery, and to evacuate a casualty no farther to the rear than his wounds demanded. This would result in a hierarchy of medical services, a chain of evacuation that carried a patient to more specialized care the farther he moved from the front.

On 2 August 1862 Maj. Gen. George B. McClellan ordered that Letterman's plan be placed into effect in the Army of the Potomac. Ambulances were to be used only for the transport of sick or wounded soldiers. Stretcher-bearers and hospital stewards were to wear distinctive insignia on their uniforms. Ambulances were to move at the head of all wagon trains, not the rear. Only medical corpsmen were to be allowed to remove the wounded from the battlefield. Although ambulances, horses, and harnesses were to be under division control, all ambulance drivers were to be under Medical Department control, trained for their work, and not allowed to assume other duties such as assisting surgeons in the field hospitals. They were also expected to be of proven good character. In March 1864 President Lincoln approved a congressional act creating a uniformed Ambulance Corps, based on Letterman's plan, for the entire Army of the United States.

Although the Ambulance Corps was disbanded at the end of the war, it had served remarkably well when it was needed. The Medical Department during the war had never overcome serious problems in the supply of medicine and the construction of field hospitals. But its numerous horse-drawn ambulances had effectively removed the wounded from the battlefields, even during the massive conflict at Gettysburg.

In the Spanish-American War and World War I, the U.S. Army had to relearn many of the medical lessons of the Civil War. By World War I ground evacuation of casualties could be accomplished by motor-driven ambulances, but the increased speed was offset to some degree by limited road access to the widely dispersed front lines in France and the Low Countries. World Wars I and II showed that automotive transport, while effective for backhauls from clearing stations to field hospitals and evacuation hospitals, was of limited value in evacuating casualties from the spot where they fell.

Early Aeromedical Evacuation

The first aeromedical evacuation occurred in the Franco-Prussian War of 1870–71. During the German seige of Paris, observation balloons flew out of the city with many bags of mail, a few high-ranking officials, and 160 casualties. Thirty-three years later at Kitty Hawk, North Carolina, Wilbur and Orville Wright proved that manned, engine-powered flight in heavier-than-air craft was actually possible. In 1908 the War Department awarded a contract to the Wright Brothers for the Army's first airplane, and in July 1909 accepted their product.

Two enterprising Army officers quickly noted the medical potential of such aircraft. At Pensacola, Florida, in the autumn of 1909, Capt. George H. R. Gosman, Medical Corps, and Lt. Albert L. Rhoades, Coast Artillery Corps, used their own money to construct a strange-looking craft in which the pilot, who was also to be a doctor, sat beside the patient. On its first powered flight the plane crashed into a tree. Lacking the funds to continue the project, Captain Gosman went to Washington to seek money from the War Department. He told one conference: "I clearly see that thousands of hours and ultimately thousands of patients would be saved through use of airplanes in air evacuation." But his audience thought the idea impractical. In May 1912 other military aviators recommended the use of air ambulances to the Secretary of War, but the War Department still thought airplanes unsuitable for such a mission. During World War I Army Aviation grew steadily, but its planes served as air ambulances only sporadically.

As they had with ground ambulances, the French pioneered the use of airplanes as ambulances. During maneuvers in 1912 an airplane helped stretcher parties on the ground locate simulated casualties. The French then designed a monoplane with a box-like structure under its fuselage for moving casualties to field hospitals. In October 1913 a French military officer reported, "We shall revolutionize war surgery if the aeroplane can be adopted as a means of transport for the wounded." During World War I the French did occasionally move the wounded by airplane, especially in November 1915 during the retreat of the Serbian Army from a combined German, Austrian, and Bulgarian attack in Albania. Although the type of aircraft used in Albania was adequate in this isolated emergency, it was hardly fit for routine use on the Western Front.

For the rest of the war the French Army gave little attention to aeromedical evacuation; they had too many casualties and too few aircraft to be concerned with it. But one French military surgeon, Dr. Eugene Chassaing, managed to keep the idea alive. When he first asked for money to build air ambulances, one officer responded, "Are there not enough dead in France today without killing the wounded in airplanes?" Despite such criticism, Chassaing acquired an old Dorland A.R. II fighter and designed a side opening that allowed two stretchers to be carried in the empty space of the fuselage behind the pilot. After several test flights of the craft, he was permitted to place six such aircraft into operation. In April 1918 two of these planes helped in the evacuations from Flanders, but the fighting grew so intense there that French higher authorities would not sanction continued use of the planes. Late in 1918 Dr. Chassaing received permission to convert sixty-four airplanes in Morocco into air ambulances, and all were used in that country in France's war against Riffian and Berber tribesmen in the Atlas mountains. The French experimented with air ambulances throughout the interwar period.

By the end of World War I the U.S. Army had also begun to reexamine its position on air ambulances. In 1920 the Army built and flew its first aircraft designed as an air ambulance, the DeHavilland DH-4A, which had space for a pilot, two litter patients, and a medical attendant. In 1924 the Army let its first contracts for air ambulances, and in the next few years it occasionally used its air ambulances to provide disaster relief to the civilian community. In April 1927, after a tornado struck the small town of Rocksprings, Texas, the Army sent eighteen DH–4 observation planes, two Douglass transports, and a Cox-Klemin XA–1 air ambulance. These planes flew in physicians and supplies to treat 200 injured citizens, some of whom the Cox-Klemin then flew out to more sophisticated medical care in San Antonio.

The decade after the war also saw the development of rotary-wing aircraft. In December 1928 the United States received from France its first sample of a rotary-wing aircraft—the autogiro, which used one motor-driven propeller for forward motion and another wind-driven propeller for vertical lift. By 1933 one U.S. manufacturer had designed an autogiro ambulance to carry a pilot and three patients, two recumbent in wire basket (Stokes) litters, and one sitting. In the December 1933 issue of the *Military Surgeon*, Lt. Col. G. P. Lawrence foresaw the military uses of this air ambulance. Since the autogiro could not hover, rough terrain, forests, and swamps would still require ground evacuation of casualties. But autogiros working from nearby landing areas could backhaul the casualties to medical stations. The advantages seemed indisputable:

Autogiros, not being limited by roads, would find more frequent opportunities to open advanced landing posts than would motor ambulances. They could maneuver and dodge behind cover so as to make hits by enemy artillery quite improbable. At night they could potter around in the dark, undisturbed by aimed enemy fire, until they accurately located the landing place, outlined by ordinary electric flash lights in the hands of the collecting company, and then land so gently that the exact estimation of altitude would be immaterial.

In 1936 the Medical Field Service School at Carlisle Barracks, Pennsylvania, tested the medical evacuation abilities of the autogiro. Though the results were promising, the Army's budgetary problems prevented funding a rotary-wing medical evacuation unit.

World War II brought the first widespread use of fixed-wing aircraft for military medical evacuation. In May 1942 the Army Medical Service activated the first U.S. aeromedical evacuation unit, the 38th Medical Air Ambulance Squadron, stationed at Fort Benning, Georgia. The war also stimulated further research on rotary-wing aircraft, both in Germany and the United States. Although Allied bombing raids destroyed the factories that the Germans intended to use for helicopter production, research and development in the United States proceeded apace. On 20 April 1942 Igor Sikorsky staged a successful flight demonstration of his helicopter. By March 1943 the Army had ordered thirty-four Sikorsky helicopters, fifteen for the U.S. Army Air Forces, fifteen for the British, and four for the U.S. Navy. These and later versions of the Sikorsky could be quickly converted to air ambulance use by attaching litters to the sides of the aircraft.

Tests at the Army Materiel Center in the summer of 1943 suggested that the helicopter could be an effective air ambulance. On 13 August 1943 the Army Surgeon stated that he intended to fill the need for a complete air evacuation service in combat zones by employing helicopters, regardless of terrain features, as the only means of evacuation from front lines to advanced airdomes. Further successful tests of the litter-bearing helicopter in November 1943 supported his decision. But helicopters were not yet abundant, and the Surgeon's plan came to nothing.

The helicopter nevertheless managed to prove its value as a device for rescue and medical evacuation from forward combat areas. In late April 1944, Lt. Carter Harman, one of the first Army Air Forces pilots trained in helicopters at the Sikorsky plant in Bridgeport, Connecticut, flew for the 1st Air Commando Force, U.S. Army Air Forces, in India. On 23 April he took one of his unit's new litter-bearing Sikorskys to pick up a stranded party with casualties about twenty-five kilometers west of Mawlu, Burma. When he returned to India he had flown the U.S. Army's first helicopter medical evacuation (medevac) mission. Soon helicopters became an item in high demand. Maj. Gen. George E. Stratemeyer, commander of the Eastern Air Command, requested six of them for the rescue of five of his pilots who had crashed in inaccessible areas and for similar rescue missions. In the spring of 1945 helicopters evacuated the sick and wounded of the 112th Regimental Combat Team and the 38th Infantry Division from remote mountain sites on the island of Luzon in the Philippines.

Most evacuation from the front lines in World War II, however, was by conventional ground ambulance. The Army Medical Service did improve its services, greatly reducing the mortality rates from those of World War I. New drugs, such as penicillin and the sulfonamides, and the stationing of major surgical facilities close to the front line, saved hundreds of thousands of lives. Airplanes evacuated over 1.5 million casualties, far more than in World War I, but this role was largely limited to transporting casualties from frontline hospitals to restorative and recuperative hospitals in the rear, rather than from site of wounding to life-saving surgical care. At the end of the war Army aeromedical evacuation still lacked a coherent system of regulations and a standing organizational base. Before it could acquire these, Army aviation would have to survive the upheaval attending the creation of the United States Air Force.

The National Security Act of 1947 established the United States Air Force as a separate military arm and at the same time stripped the Army of most of its aircraft, leaving it only about two hundred light planes and helicopters. The general mission of Army aviation was limited to furthering ground combat operations in forward areas of the battlefield, a mission that fortunately encompassed responsibility for emergency aeromedical evacuation from the front. However, when the Korean War opened three years later, the Army Medical Service still had no helicopter ambulance units.

The Korean War

The Korean War resulted in a rapid, new buildup of American military forces, which had been precipitously reduced after World War II. This was no less true for the Army Medical Service than for other U.S. military agencies. At first, in July 1950, only a single evacuation hospital and one Mobile Army Surgical Hospital (MASH) supported all U.S. forces in Korea. By the end of the year these medical resources had grown to four mobile surgical hospitals, three field hospitals, two 500-bed station hospitals, one evacuation hospital, and the Swedish Red Cross Hospital near Pusan. The medical buildup was timely, for between 7 July and 31 December 1950 United Nations forces suffered nearly 62,000 casualties. Medical support expanded even further in 1951.

The Korean War resulted in the first systematic use of helicopters for evacuation of casualties from the battlefield. The rugged, often mountainous terrain and the poor, insecure road network in wartime Korea made overland movement extremely difficult. Transport of wounded and injured ground troops from the front line rearward by litter bearers or jeep ambulances seriously aggravated the patient's condition, caused deepened shock, and often produced fatal complications. Just before the war broke out Lt. Gen. Walton Walker, the Eighth U.S. Army, Korea (EUSAK) commander, told his senior surgeon that in event of hostilities he wanted mobile surgical hospitals placed as close to the front lines as possible. During the war the mobile surgical hospitals, stationed from five to forty kilometers behind the front, served as the main destination of ground and air ambulances bringing casualties from clearing stations at the front. Most of the casualties arrived in ground ambulances, but 10 to 20 percent were brought by helicopters. The Air Force and Navy also used helicopters for medical evacuation, but the Army's helicopter ambulance detachments carried the great majority of the war's helicopter evacuees.

The Air Force, however, pioneered the use of helicopter ambulances in Korea. In July 1950, just after the war broke out, Helicopter Detachment F of the Air Force's Third Air Rescue Squadron began to receive requests for evacuation of forward Army casualties in areas inaccessible to ground vehicles. Col. Chauncey E. Dovell, the Eighth Army Surgeon, arranged a test of the Third Air Rescue Squadron's H-5 helicopters in the courtyard of the Taequ

Teachers' College. On 3 August he and Capt. Oscar N. Tibbetts, the squadron's commander, met at the college and examined one of the H–5's. A Stokes litter fit into the compartment of the H–5 very well, but the handles of the standard Army litter had to be cut off. With two patients and Colonel Dovell on board, the H–5 lifted off, easily cleared the surrounding telephone poles and buildings, and returned for a perfect landing. Colonel Dovell asked to see a long flight, so the pilot flew him and the two patients out to the 8054th Evacuation Hospital at Pusan, 100 kilometers away. On 10 August, at Colonel Dovell's request, Lt. Gen. Earle E. Partridge, commander of the Fifth Air Force, authorized the use of these and other Air Force helicopters for frontline evacuations. The Air Force continued to evacuate the Army's frontline casualties until the end of the year, allowing the Army time to organize and ship to Korea its own helicopter detachments.

Late in the year the Army deployed four helicopter detachments to Korea. These units, each authorized four H–13 Sioux helicopters, contained no medical personnel, but were under the operational control of the EUSAK Surgeon. Each was attached to a separate mobile surgical hospital, with a primary mission of aeromedical evacuation. The crewmembers drew their rations and quarters from the MASH, and their aircraft parts and service from wherever they could be found. The 2d Helicopter Detachment became operational on 1 January 1951; the 3d, later in January; and the 4th, in March. The 1st Helicopter Detachment, which arrived in February, never became operational because commanders transferred all of its aircraft to other nonmedical units. At the height of the Korean conflict the three operational helicopter detachments controlled only eleven aircraft. But by the end of the war they had evacuated about 17,700 casualties, supplemented by a considerable number of medevac missions performed by nonmedical helicopters organic to division light air sections and helicopters of Army cargo transportation companies. Marine and Air Force helicopters had also made a sizable number of frontline evacuations.

The independence and therefore the value of the air ambulance units increased after the introduction of detailed standard operating procedures. Typical of those adopted by the detachments was the list that Lt. Col. Carl T. Dubuy, commander of the 1st Mobile Army Surgical Hospital, drew up in early February 1951. Evacuation requests were to be made only for patients with serious wounds, or where surface transport would seriously worsen a casualty's injuries. The helicopters would be used strictly for medical evacuation and reconnaissance, and would not be used for command, administrative, or tactical missions. Each request for a helicopter was to include a clear and careful reading of the coordinates of the pickup site. The ground commander was to try to find the lowest pickup site around, to ease the strain on the minimally powered H–13 helicopters that performed the bulk of medical evacuations in Korea. A request was not to be made for a landing zone subject to hostile fire; if trouble did develop, the men on the ground were to wave off the helicopter. Dubuy recommended the use of colored panels to form a cross to mark the pickup site, and he also favored some indicator of wind direction and velocity, such as grass fire. He suggested that if the helicopter flew past the pickup zone without recognizing it, the soldiers on the ground should fire flares or smoke grenades to attract the pilot's attention. (The aircraft had no radios.) Colonel Dubuy sent these recommended procedures to the commanding general of the 7th Infantry Division, which the 1st Mobile Army Surgical Hospital then supported, but the division afforded the list only a haphazard distribution.

In January 1951 all four pilots of the 2d Helicopter Detachment took part in a mission that, although it violated the precept that helicopters would not be flown within range of enemy weapons, saved several lives. On the morning of 13 January, Capt. Albert C. Sebourn of the 2d Detachment received an urgent request for air evacuation from a unit at a schoolhouse surrounded by a large Chinese Communist force near Choksong-ni. The unit was a Special Activities Group (SAG), an elite, battalion-size organization of airborne and ranger-qualified soldiers. Their only defensive perimeter was the border of the one acre schoolyard. A MASH doctor had been asking for a ride in a helicopter. Sebourn put him in the right seat and then flew to the coordinates of the request. After landing in the schoolyard, Sebourn shut down the helicopter. As soon as he and the doctor climbed out, a mortar round landed near the right side of the helicopter, damaging it but not injuring anyone. Both men ran into the schoolhouse, where the commander of the SAG unit explained that he had numerous casualties and wanted the helicopter to bring in ammunition on its return flights from the hospital. When Sebourn tried to restart his aircraft, he found that the battery was dead; he and the doctor stayed at the school overnight.

When Sebourn did not return to the 2d Detachment's base after several hours, Capt. Joseph W. Hely checked back through Eighth Army channels. The request had been quite old when the 2d Detachment received it: it had been routed through Tokyo. Eighth Army asked Hely whether he would fly ammunition out to the beleaguered force, and he assented. With ammunition in both his aircraft's litter pods, he tried to fly out, but heavy snowfall made him postpone the flight until the weather improved. Next morning, when he reached the area, he noticed tracers from enemy machine guns trying to shoot him down. He spiraled down into the schoolyard, unloaded the ammunition, gave the battery in Sebourn's helicopter a boost, and then loaded two patients in his own craft. He spiraled out to escape the enemy fire again and Sebourn followed him.

Later that day two other 2d Detachment pilots joined Hely in two more flights to the schoolyard, carrying food and ammunition to the SAG unit and casualties back to the hospital. Enemy ground fire harassed each entry and exit at the schoolyard. On leaving the school for the last time just before darkness, Hely radioed an Air Force fighter and marked the perimeter for its strike. The next morning the 2d Detachment made a final evacuation from the schoolyard before the SAG unit withdrew. Captains Hely and Sebourn won Distinguished Flying Crosses for their work.

The communications net used to route and obtain approval of a ground commander's request for such a medevac mission was laborious at best, especially early in the war. The request usually originated at a casualty collecting station in the field or at a battalion aid station. Then it was relayed by radio or telephone to the division surgeon, then to the corps surgeon, and finally to the Eighth Army Surgeon, who decided if the mission was valid. If he approved, the approval passed back down the ladder to the helicopter detachment attached to the hospital supporting the corps area. This process often delayed a mission for hours, and sometimes it led to a cancellation because the casualty had already died. Some procedures, though, helped speed the response time of the helicopters. Stationing a mobile surgical hospital and its helicopter detachment close to the front line, usually some ten to forty kilometers behind it, reduced the response time. Eventually the Eighth Army Surgeon ceded mission approval authority to the corps surgeons, who had direct communications with the mobile surgical hospitals, thereby eliminating one level in the three-tiered approval structure.

To improve the communications and speed the response, the helicopter detachments began the practice of siting their aircraft in the field at clearing stations near the tactical headquarters just behind the front lines. These one-aircraft field standbys ensured ready and rapid transportation of the critically wounded to mobile surgical hospitals. But this solution produced another problem. Since the helicopters themselves carried no radios, an aircraft that was field-sited with a combat unit that had a poor radio linkup with other combat units in the Corps zone could not respond rapidly to sudden fighting in other areas. The absence of radios in the aircraft also precluded any air-ground communication and made necessary the use of smoke signals and hand gestures to ensure the safe completion of a mission. In the first months of the war not even the detachment headquarters had radios. When available, they helped immensely by freeing the detachments from their dependence on Army switchboards and landlines.

Several times division commanders tried to obtain the assignment of helicopters to specific combat units for evacuation missions (direct support). For instance, the 3d Infantry Division, with an indorsement from I Corps, requested its own air ambulance; I Corps wanted to give each division its own air ambulance. But EUSAK headquarters denied the request because there were not enough helicopters to provide such individualized coverage, and the current area and standby coverage was working adequately.

Many other problems in this new system proved intractable. The most serious came from the constant need to repair the helicopter. The sluggishness of the Air Force, the Army's aviation procurement agency, in meeting Army aviation's supply needs created a backlog of requests for helicopter parts and components. Just as American industry at the start of World War II was unable to fill all the Army's requests for airplanes, so at the start of the Korean War it was not geared for helicopter production. The fine tolerances required because of the many rotating and revolving parts in a helicopter, and the limited commercial potential for the craft, made American aircraft manufacturers reluctant to devote their resources to such a chancy investment. When production did increase, a serious problem arose in transporting the vast quantities of war materiel from the States to Korea. All of these problems adversely affected the supply of spare parts, fuel, and even aircraft. By late 1952 the eleven air ambulance helicopters in Korea had to compete with about 635 other Army nonmedical helicopters for whatever resources the American aircraft industry could provide.

Parts shortages in the field accounted for the loss of much valuable flying time in all Army aviation units in Korea, more so than any other problem. In a three month period in 1952 the 8193d Army Unit lost about one-third of its potential aircraft days because of parts shortages. This resulted in lives lost because the unit was unable to respond to all evacuation requests. The 8193d commander, Capt. Emil R. Day, requested that a fifth helicopter be assigned to each of the MASH helicopter detachments, but this was not done. In allocating parts the Air Force favored its own fighters and bombers over the Army helicopters. Supply personnel in the States seemed to have little awareness of the cost in human life of returning supply requests for editorial changes, explanations of excess requirements, and "proper" item descriptions. Harry S. Pack, in an evaluation of the problems of helicopter evacuation in Korea, aptly criticized the support system:

> The basic concept of the employment of the helicopter in the Army...is its increased speed over other forms of transport currently in use in the movement of personnel and materiel. Therefore, it is only logical that the entire helicopter program, including maintenance and supply procedures, should follow the same philosophy of speed and mobility to ensure receiving maximum value from the helicopter.

The focal point of these supply problems was the Bell Aircraft Corporation's H–13 Sioux helicopter, which performed almost all aeromedical evacuations in Korea. Powered by a Franklin engine, it sported a large plexiglass bubble over the top and front of the cockpit. It could transport a pilot and one passenger, and two patients on external litters. Although Bell Aircraft sent some of its test pilots to Korea to help the Army pilots obtain maximum performance from the H–13, the aircraft simply had not been designed for medical evacuations in mountainous terrain. The H–13's standard fuel capacity could not keep the aircraft aloft the two or more hours that many evacuation flights took. The pilots had to either fuel at the pickup site or carry extra fuel in five-gallon cans. The cans could be carried in the cockpit or, more safely, strapped to the litter pods and left at the pickup site. Also, since the battery in the H–13 was not powerful enough to guarantee restarting the aircraft without a boost, the pilots often practiced "hot refueling" in the field. Although dangerous, the practice seemed safer than being unable to restart the aircraft near the front line.

Because the H–13D's the pilots flew had no instrument or cockpit lights and no gyroscopic attitude indicators, most evacuation missions took place in daylight. But extreme emergencies sometimes prompted the pilots to complete a night mission by flying with a flashlight held between their legs to illuminate the flight instruments. The expedient barely worked, because the bouncing, flickering beam of the flashlight often produced a blinding glare.

When the first Army aeromedical unit in Korea, the 2d Helicopter Detachment, arrived at the end of 1950 and put its equipment in working order, it still could not declare itself operational, because the H–13D's lacked litter platforms, attaching points on the helicopters, or even litters. The unit quickly received permission to fit platforms on the skid assemblies so that litters could be mounted on either side of the fuselage. When the EUSAK Aviation Section failed to obtain litters for the detachment, its commander, Captain Sebourn, turned to the Navy hospital ship in the Inchon Harbor. The Navy people gave him eight of their metal, basket-like Stokes litters. The detachment then had to find covers for them to protect the patients from the elements and secure them to the pod. Lt. Joseph L. Bowler took the litters to Taegu, found some heavy steel wire, and then had a welder at a maintenance company fashion a lid with a plexiglass window that could be attached to the litter, enclosing the patient's upper body. Next, both the lid and the litter were covered with aircraft fabric and several coats of dope. This laborious process required repeated painting and drying in the cold, sleet, and snow of the Korean winter.

The improvised pods and litters proved far from ideal. Loading and unloading the patient was an awkward process, since he had to be taken from the standard Army field litter, lifted onto a blanket, and then placed into the Stokes litter. Some patients with certain types of casts, splints, and dressings could not be moved by helicopter at all because of the confined space of the Stokes litter. The pilots and mechanics improvised heating for the inside of these litters by fabricating manifold shrouds and ducting warm air off the manifolds into the litters. Even so, the patients had to be covered with mountain sleeping bags or plastic bags. If the manifold heat were used on one litter only, excess warm air escaped near the hose connection; but if heat were turned on both litters, there was not enough for either. The problem partly stemmed from the plastic cover; it lay directly on the patient and did not allow the heat to circulate properly. So the detachments worked with a maintenance company and a Bell Aircraft technical representative, constructing a three-quarter length cover of fabric-covered tubing that could be joined to the original head cover. It served as a windbreak and gave space for the heat to circulate over the patient's lower body.

In July 1951 a new litter mount, manufactured by Bell Aircraft for the H–13, reached Korea. These greatly improved mounts accommodated a standard Army field litter, eliminating the need to transfer a patient to a Stokes litter before placing him in the pod. Unfortunately the covers that Bell manufactured for the new mount were usually torn up by the slipstream after just thirty days of use. The detachments improvised a canvas cover from pup tent shelter halves; when used with the zipper and snaps from the Bell cover, it proved far superior to the original in that it had a long service life and kept water from seeping through onto the patient. The men of the detachments used their own money and Korean labor to produce an ample supply of covers.

Even with the improved pods, the external mounting and the absence of a medical corpsman on the aircraft produced another difficulty. Pilots began to notice that many of the casualties needed transfusions before being moved to a mobile surgical hospital. In cold weather an in-flight transfusion with the fluids stored outside the aircraft risked deepening the patient's shock as the fluid temperature dropped. At first the pilots would wait the thirty or forty-five minutes necessary for a transfusion before departing with a patient. Then Lt. Col. James M. Brown, commander of the 8063d Mobile Surgical Hospital, devised a method for en route transfusions of plasma or whole blood. A bottle of blood or plasma was attached to the inside wall of the cockpit within reach of the pilot. Needles and plasma would be arranged before departure, and during flight the pilot could monitor the fluid flow through the tubes extending to the litter pods. A rubber bulb could be used to regulate pressure to the bottle. This modification was approved for all medical helicopters in the theater, and Bell Aircraft also incorporated it in all its D-model aircraft.

Since the Eighth Army possessed only thirty-two H–13's by May

1951, use of the valuable craft had to be closely monitored and restricted. A recurring problem was that ground commanders sometimes requested helicopters more as a convenience than as a necessity. To prevent this, the EUSAK Surgeon on 23 June 1951 disseminated a statement that the role of helicopter evacuation was only to provide immediate evacuation of nontransportable and critically ill or injured patients who needed surgical or medical care not available at forward medical facilities. This statement was given wider distribution than had Colonel Dubuy's in February and it noticeably reduced the number of unnecessary missions.

The detachments offered their service to all of the fighting units involved in the United Nations effort in Korea. At first glance it seemed that the language barrier would make many of these missions extremely difficult. But the lack of air-ground communications helped in this respect, for it precluded any attempt whatsoever at oral communication between pilots and ground commanders. Most pilots found that universal sign language usually sufficed to transmit any information necessary to complete an evacuation. In September 1951 one of the pilots received a request to pick up two wounded men from a Turkish brigade. The pilot recalled:

When I got to the spot designated I couldn't find anybody. I was circling around when a Turkish observation plane buzzed me. He led me to a wooded area on a mountain top where the Turks had dug in. The trees were too high to permit a landing. It looked pretty hopeless because I couldn't communicate with them. Finally, I went in close until the rotor blades of the helicopter brushed the tops of the trees. The Turks got the pitch. They chopped down enough of the trees so that I could land on a ridge. I sat down and the Chinese began tossing mortar shells at me. But I got the two wounded Turks out.

Enemy ground resistance to air ambulances in Korea never became a severe problem, as it did later in Vietnam. Few landing zones were subject to enemy small arms fire, but many were within range of enemy artillery and mortars. Although the pilots generally stayed out of landing zones under enemy fire, several had more than one encounter with Communist weapons. At one point early in the war a company of the 7th Infantry Division was fighting in the area known as the Iron Triangle. In assaulting an enemy-held slope, two of its soldiers were seriously wounded by the Chinese. A request for an air ambulance quickly made its way to the 4th Helicopter Detachment, stationed with the 8076th Mobile Surgical Hospital at Chunchon. CBS correspondent Robert Pierpoint was there and had received permission to fly with the detachment. Three minutes after the call came in, a pilot and Pierpoint flew north toward the pickup site. The men on the ground put out colored panels to mark a landing zone on a nearby paddy, while others tried to bring the casualties down from the hill. Thirty minutes after the call went out, the helicopter landed at the marked position. The pilot and Pierpoint got out. Just as the litter bearers made it down the hill, Chinese mortars from across the valley opened up on the paddy. A mortar round came in, hit about thirty feet from the helicopter tail, and sent the Americans scrambling up the hill. The company commander called an artillery battalion 6,000 yards to the rear, and had them knock out the Chinese mortar positions.

The pilots, Pierpoint, and the litter bearers returned to the helicopter and loaded the casualties. Not waiting to check for damage, the pilot climbed into the smoke-filled cockpit. He could hardly see the instruments, but, as soon as Pierpoint jumped in, they made a maximum power takeoff. They landed at the hospital at 2120, reading their aircraft instruments with a flashlight one of the men at the paddy had given them.

In another respect, Korea was worse than Vietnam: the ambulance crews sometimes had to contend with enemy aircraft. Although the U.S. Air Force destroyed most of the North Korean aircraft early in the conflict, the entrance of the Chinese Communists into the war in December 1950 brought fast and powerful enemy jet fighters to Korea. A few medical helicopters did encounter fire from North Korean Yak fighters, but the Americans outmaneuvered the faster jets and escaped damage.

Apart from frontline evacuations, air ambulance detachments also flew a few other medical support missions. By the second year of the war they routinely transported whole blood to the mobile surgical hospitals. This proved valuable because the whole blood tended to break down prematurely or clot when carried by surface vehicles over the rough Korean roads. The faster means of transport also allowed blood storage and refrigeration to be centralized rather than dispersed close to the front. The helicopters backhauled some critical patients from the mobile surgical hospitals to airstrips for further evacuation to one of the general hospitals in Japan. Sometimes they even backhauled patients to hospital ships along the coast, such as the Navy's hospital ship *Consolation* and the Danish *Jutlandia*, which were equipped for helicopter landings. Since fixed-wing cargo planes flew all casualties bound for Japan, the hospital ships remained anchored as floating hospitals off Korea rather than act as ferries.

Most detachment pilots also tried to make the life of the frontline soldiers as tolerable as they could. Besides medical supplies and ammunition, the pilots often took beer, ice cream, and sodas to the front. The sight of the helicopter coming in for a landing in the blistering Korean summer with the pilot wearing only his boots, a red baseball cap, and swimming trunks, and then unloading these otherwise unobtainable luxuries, did much to boost the morale of the combat soldiers.

Apart from yielding a great deal of practical experience, the Korean War furthered aeromedical evacuation by convincing the Army that the helicopter ambulances deserved a permanent organization. When the war broke out, the Army Medical Service commanded neither helicopters nor pilots, and its leaders were not committed to furthering aeromedical evacuation. In Korea the Eighth Army soon acquired virtually complete operational control of the helicopter detachments charged with a mission of medical evacuation. But the Surgeon General wanted to have the detachments made organic to the Medical Service, to have an organization within the Office of the Surgeon General capable of directing and administering the aviation resources, and to have medical personnel rather than aviators from other branches of the Army piloting the aircraft.

The Surgeon General achieved his first goal with the publication on 20 August 1952 of TO&E 8–500A, which provided for an air ambulance detachment of seven officers, twenty-one enlisted men, and five utility helicopters. The first such unit was the 53d Medical Detachment (Helicopter Ambulance), activated at Brooke Army Medical Center, Fort Sam Houston, San Antonio, Texas, on 15 October 1952. In Korea, meanwhile, the ambulance units were transfered from the administrative command of the Eighth Army Flight Detachment to that of the Eighth Army Surgeon.

By the end of the war the Surgeon General also succeeded in achieving his second goal of creating a special aviation section in his office. On 30 June 1952 the Chief of Staff of the Army directed the Chairman of the Materiel Review Board to evaluate the Army helicopter program. In accordance with the Board's recommendation, the Chief of Staff on 17 October 1952 directed the assistant chiefs of staff and the various Army branch chiefs to set up their own agencies to supervise and coordinate aviation within each office. The Surgeon General's Office was charged with coordination of all planning, operations, personnel staffing, and supply of Army aviation used in the Medical Service. On 6 November the office established the Army Aviation Section within the Hospitalization and Operations Branch, Medical Plans and Operations Division. On the advice of the new section, the Surgeon General recommended that "...all aircraft designed, developed, or accepted for the Army (regardless of its intended primary use) be chosen with a view toward potential use as air ambulances to accommodate a maximum number of standard litters." This advice was followed in 1955 when the Army held a design competition for a new multipurpose utility helicopter. The winner of the competition, the Bell Aircraft Corporation's prototype of the UH–1 Iroquois ("Huey"), eventually became the Army's standard ambulance helicopter in the Vietnam War.

During the Korean War the Surgeon General also tried to place

Medical Service Corps (MSC) pilots in the cockpits of the Army's air ambulances.[2] But he did not succeed until shortly after the armistice in 1953. From early 1951 on, the Surgeon General had advocated training some MSC officers as aviators, and in the spring of 1952 the regulations governing Army aviation were amended to allow MSC personnel to become pilots. A quota of twenty-five MSC officers, mostly second lieutenants, was set for flight training in October. None of the current MSC officers had ever been helicopter pilots, although a few had had some aviation training. By early July, fifty-three applications for the slots had been received, but only seventeen applicants were qualified. Eight MSC officers began flight training in October, and one washed out before graduation. The other seven graduated on 28 February 1953. In September the Surgeon General's office requested and received a standing quota of ten MSC officers per month for attendance at the Army Aviation School at Fort Sill, Oklahoma. By 1 October the Medical Service had twenty-four officer pilots and soon received five more by transfer from other branches. None had flown in Korea before the armistice in July.

After the Korean War the Surgeon General's Office applied itself to assessing the potential of helicopter ambulances in future conflicts. In particular, Lt. Col. Spurgeon H. Neel, Jr., in a number of medical and aviation journals, publicized and promoted the Army's air ambulances. The Korean experience, he realized, could not serve as an infallible guide to the use of helicopters in other types of wars and different geographical regions, but it certainly showed that helicopters had made possible at least a modification of the first links in Letterman's chain of evacuation. A superior communications system would allow a well-equipped and well-staffed ambulance to land at or near the site of the wounding, making much ground evacuation unnecessary. If the patient's condition could be stabilized briefly, it might prove helpful to use the speed of the helicopter to evacuate the patient farther to the rear, to more complete medical facilities than those provided at a rudimentary division clearing station. Triage might be carried out better at a hospital than in the field. But the Korean War and the concurrent French struggle in Indochina had afforded only limited, imperfect tests of helicopter medical evacuation. The potential was obvious, but not fully proven.

---

[2]At this time the Army Medical Service consisted of six corps: Medical, Dental, Veterinary Army Nurse, Women's Medical Specialists, and the Medical Service Corps, which provided a variety of administrative and technical services.

CHAPTER II

Birth Of A Tradition

The lay of the land and the guerrilla nature of Viet Cong warfare in South Vietnam demanded that the American forces stationed there from the early 1960s through March 1973 again use the medical helicopter. In a country of mountains, jungles, and marshy plains, with few passable roads and serviceable railroads, the allied forces waged a frontless war against a seldom seen enemy. Even more than in Korea, helicopter evacuation proved to be both valuable and dangerous.

South Vietnam consists of three major geographic features. A coastal plain, varying in width from fifteen to forty kilometers, extends along most of the 1,400 kilometers of the coast. This plain abuts the second feature—the southeastern edge of the Annamite Mountain Chain, known in South Vietnam as the Central Highlands, which run from the northern border along the old Demilitarized Zone south to within eighty kilometers of Saigon. The Central Highlands are mostly steep-sloped, sharp-crested mountains varying in height from 5,000 to 8,000 feet, covered with tangled jungles and broken by many narrow passes. The southern third of the country consists almost entirely of an arable delta.

These three geographical features helped shape the four military zones of South Vietnam. The northern zone, or I Corps Zone, which ran from the Demilitarized Zone down to Kontum and Binh Dinh provinces, consisted almost entirely of high mountains and dense jungles. At several points the Annamites cut the narrow coastal plain and extend to the South China Sea. II Corps Zone ran from I Corps Zone south to the southern foothills of the Central Highlands, about one hundred kilometers north of Saigon. It consisted of a long stretch of the coastal plain, the highest portion of the Central Highlands, and the Kontum and Darlac Plateaus. III Corps Zone ran from II Corps Zone southwest to a line forty kilometers below the capital, Saigon. This was an intermediate geographic region, containing the southern foothills of the Central Highlands; a few large, dry plains; some thick, triple-canopy jungle along the Cambodian border; and the northern stretches of the delta formed by the Mekong River to the south. IV Corps Zone consisted almost entirely of this delta, which has no forests except for dense mangrove swamps at the southernmost tip and forested areas just north and southeast of Saigon. Seldom more than twenty feet above sea level, the delta is covered with rice fields separated by earthen dikes. During the rainy season the paddies are marshy, making helicopter landings and vehicular troop transport extremely difficult. Hamlets straddle the rivers and canals, and larger villages (up to 10,000 people) and cities lie at the junctions of the waterways. Bamboo brakes and tropical trees grow around the villages and usually extend from 50 to 300 meters back on either side of the canal or hamlet.

The entire country lies below the Tropic of Cancer, between the 8th and 17th parallels. The climate is generally hot and humid the year round. In winter the country lies under a high pressure system that causes a dry season in the south. In the summer, however, rains fall heavily, varying from torrential downpours to steady mists. The northern region of South Vietnam has the most rain, averaging 128 inches, while the Saigon region averages 80 inches. In the northern region and the Central Highlands, where most of the fighting by U.S. troops during the war occurred, dense fog and low clouds often grounded all aircraft. About ten times a year, usually between July and November, typhoons blow in from the South China Sea, soaking South Vietnam with heavy rains and lashing it with fierce winds.

Although the climate and terrain exacerbated the technical problems of medical evacuation by helicopter in South Vietnam, the air ambulance pilots who worked there worried as much or more about the dangers that stemmed from the enemy's frequent use of guerrilla tactics. The Viet Cong were wily, elusive, and intensely motivated. They usually had no respect for the red crosses on the doors of the air ambulance helicopters. Likely to be annihilated in a large-scale, head-on clash with the immense firepower of American troops, they usually struck only in raids and ambushes of American and South Vietnamese patrols. To perform their missions the air ambulance pilots often had to fly into areas subject to intense enemy small arms fire. Later in the war the pilots encountered more formidable obstacles, such as Russian- and Chinese-made ground-to-air missiles. No air ambulance pilot could depend on a ground commander's assurance that a pickup zone was secure. Mortar and small arms fire often found a zone just as the helicopter touched down. Enemy soldiers were known to patiently hide for hours around an ambushed patrol, looking for the inevitable rescue helicopter.

In these conditions the modern techniques of aeromedical evacuation developed and matured. The obstacles of mountain, jungle, and floodplain could be overcome only by helicopters. The frontless nature of the war also made necessary the helicopter for medical evacuation. Air ambulance units found ever wider employment as the helicopter—used both as a fighting machine and as a transport vehicle—came to dominate many phases of the war.

The Struggle Begins

In 1961 President John F. Kennedy took the first of a number of measures that over the next four years drew the United States deep into the stormy politics of Southeast Asia. In May, Kennedy publicly repeated a pledge, first made by President Dwight D. Eisenhower in 1954, of U.S. support for the government of the Republic of Vietnam. Kennedy had the Department of State adopt a less demanding diplomacy in its dealings with the troubled regime of President Ngo Dinh Diem. The department tried to coax Diem into making urgently needed political, economic, and military reforms, but he dallied, and the Viet Cong summer campaign of 1961 further weakened his tenuous hold on the country. U.S. officials knew that he was losing control rapidly when, in September, the rebels captured a provincial capital only ninety kilometers from Saigon.

President Kennedy now believed that he had to decide whether to watch a U.S. ally collapse or to find some way of helping Diem fight the Viet Cong. In October 1961 Gen. Maxwell D. Taylor, the President's personal military adviser, and Dr. Walt W. Rostow, one of the President's aides, recommended that the United States commit some of its combat troops to Diem's defense. But Kennedy turned down this proposal. Instead he persuaded Diem to agree to a program of broad reforms, in return for the deployment of more U.S. military advisers and military equipment to support the combat operations of the Army of the Republic of Vietnam (ARVN).

On 11 December 1961 Saigon saw the arrival of the first direct U.S. military support for South Vietnam — the 8th Transportation Company from Fort Bragg, North Carolina, and the 57th Transportation Company from Fort Lewis, Washington. Both were light helicopter units. The two companies consisted of 400 pilots, crews, and technicians, with thirty-three U.S. Army H–21 Shawnee helicopters. The aircraft carrier that brought them, the U.S.S. *Core,* also brought four T–28 single-engine, propeller aircraft en route to the Vietnamese National Air Force (VNAF). With its deck towering over hundreds of nearby junks, the *Core* edged up the Saigon River to a pier in front of the Majestic Hotel. Thousands of Vietnamese lined the riverbanks and watched the start of a new phase in the war dividing their country.

In January and February 1962 two more helicopter companies, the 93d Transportation and the 18th Aviation, arrived in Saigon. The city struggled to find room for several thousand personnel from helicopter companies, Air Force training groups, engineer detachments, the Seventh Fleet, and sundry advisory units. The South Vietnamese Army, equipped with American armored personnel carriers and backed by the new American helicopters, began to show a more aggressive spirit. Accompanied by U.S. advisers, it attacked previously inviolate Viet Cong strongholds, such as War Zone D north of Saigon, and the U Minh Forest in the southern Mekong Delta.

The First Air Ambulance Unit in Vietnam

Despite their early successes in 1962, both the South Vietnamese and their American advisers suffered growing numbers of casualties. By the end of the year the medical part of the Vietnam troop list had expanded to encompass units able to provide a full range of medical services for a planned eight thousand U.S. military personnel. In Washington, Maj. Gen. James H. Forsee, Chief of Professional Services at Walter Reed, and Col. James T. McGibony, Chief of the Medical Plans and Operations Division, assured the Surgeon General that the medical units assigned to Vietnam would supply fully integrated health care. Forsee and McGibony designated the first Army medical units that would go to Vietnam to support the U.S. buildup: the 8th Field Hospital; medical detachments for dental, thoracic, orthopedic, and neurosurgical care; and the 57th Medical Detachment (Helicopter Ambulance). Arriving in April 1962, the 57th remained there throughout the next eleven years of American military involvement in that country.

This long ordeal began for the air ambulance pilots and crews in late February 1962, when Headquarters of the U.S. Second Army ordered the 57th, stationed at Fort George Meade, Maryland, for a permanent assignment to the U.S. Army, Pacific. A frenzied logistical effort began. Since the 57th was not authorized a cook, the commander, Capt. John Temperelli, Jr., obtained a six months supply of C-rations. Since they had no survival equipment, the unit's men hastily made up their kits from local stores. The typical kit, stored in a parachute bag, contained a machete, canned water, C-rations, a lensatic compass, extra ammunition, a signaling mirror, and sundry items the men thought they might need in a crisis. When they arrived in Vietnam in late April, the pilots had five "Hueys," as their UH-1 helicopters were nicknamed. Along with the 8th Field Hospital and the other medical detachments, the 57th set itself up in the seaside town of Nha Trang, 320 kilometers northeast of overcrowded Saigon. The assignment of U.S. Army medical units to Nha Trang prevented a worsening of the logistics problem in Saigon, but it placed medical support far from most of the U.S. military units in the country.

On its first mission the 57th evacuated a U.S. Army captain advising the ARVN forces. An evacuation request came on 12 May from Tuy Hoa, sixty-five kilometers up the coast from Nha Trang. The captain, suffering from an extremely high fever, was carried to the 8th

Field Hospital. Soon after, the 57th began to evacuate ARVN soldiers as well, even from combat. Although the U.S. Military Assistance Advisory Group (MAAG) prohibited the 57th from evacuating Vietnamese soldiers and civilians, Captain Temperelli found this policy to be unrealistic. He had to work closely with local Vietnamese officials to set up designated evacuation sites in secure areas and to improve the communication nets that relayed the 57th's evacuation requests. Forced to use the ARVN radio channels, the 57th was obliged to honor requests for evacuation of Vietnamese casualties. In the years ahead the air ambulances carried the wounded of all nationalities, even those of the enemy.

As yet, however, the 57th was a new unit, little known, and with little to do. It spent most of that summer sitting in Nha Trang, unable to get to the fighting. By the end of June the detachment had evacuated only twelve American and fourteen ARVN personnel. In an attempt to increase his range of action, Temperelli assigned two of his Hueys to Qui Nhon, another coastal town some 160 kilometers to the north. Neither base had refueling sites in its area. The radius of action from each was only 140 kilometers, and most of the fighting was at least 200 kilometers to the south. Hoping to add an extra fifty-five minutes flying time to each helicopter, Temperelli asked for permission to replace the unnecessary cockpit heaters with auxiliary fuel cells; but he never received approval for the change. He also tried to have the helicopters' JP–4 fuel stored in certain critical inland areas, but was only partially successful. He could also obtain no favorable response to his several requests for permission to move the unit to Saigon or the Delta.

Early in July 1962 all commanders of U.S. Army aviation units in South Vietnam met in Saigon to discuss the possibility of the extensive use of Army aviation in support of South Vietnamese counterinsurgency operations. Briefing officers told the commanders that greater American military involvement would probably require Army aviation to assume many duties formerly assigned to armor, ground transport, and the infantry. Captain Temperelli left this conference angered that, in spite of the predicted growth of Army aviation in Vietnam, the Army Medical Service had so far furnished only limited resources to his unit. The reluctance of the Vietnamese Air Force to respond to many evacuation requests convinced him that the burden of medical evacuation in this war would have to fall on U.S. Army helicopter ambulance units. Yet so far the Surgeon General had sent no representative to the 57th to see what its problems were.

In fact, the logistics problems of the 57th were only a small part of the shortages that hindered all Army aviation units in the first years of the war. Deficiencies and excesses in the authorized lists of equipment too often appeared only after units were committed to combat. Many of the aviation units carried unnecessary heaters and winter clothing with them to Vietnam simply because the standard equipment list called for them. Red tape compounded equipment problems. At first the aviation units sent their orders for parts directly to the U.S. Army on Okinawa, but Okinawa often returned the paperwork for corrections to comply with directives that the forces in Vietnam had never heard of. Only after several months of logistical chaos did the Army Support Group, Vietnam (USASGV) begin to coordinate the requisition of parts.

In this first year of operations Army supply depots in the Pacific could fill only three-fourths of the aviation orders from Vietnam. This problem arose partly from the unusual role of the Army aviation units there. Army helicopters used in support of ARVN operations flew far more hours and wore out much faster than peacetime supply estimates provided for. By November 1962 the Army had thirteen aviation units flying 199 aircraft of eight types at ten places in Vietnam. Multiple bases for several units added to the units' supply needs.

Since the 57th Medical Detachment had the only UH–1's in Vietnam so far, it could draw on no pool of replacement parts. Instead, it had to cannibalize one of its own helicopters to keep the others flying. When Gen. Paul D. Harkins, commander of the Military Assistance Command, Vietnam (MACV), and Gen. Earle G. Wheeler, Army Chief of Staff, visited Nha Trang in August 1962, they saw two of the 57th's UH–1's sitting on a ramp, with no rotor blades. The 57th had no spares.

Then combat aviation units began to demand the 57th's few remaining parts. In November, feeling confident after an influx of new infantry equipment from the United States, the South Vietnamese Army planned a large scale combat assault into the "Iron Triangle," a Viet Cong stronghold northwest of Saigon. Armed Huey UH–1's were to cover the CH–21's carrying ARVN troops to the landing zones. Since several of the Hueys had bad tail rotor gear boxes and faulty starter generators, the 57th received instructions to bring all its starter generators to Saigon. Plainly, the unit's craft were about to be cannibalized.

To head off the danger, Temperelli accompanied the generators to Saigon and reported to Brig. Gen. Joseph W. Stilwell, commander of the Army Support Group, Vietnam. Noting that the absence of the generators on the 57th's aircraft would leave South Vietnam without air evacuation coverage, Temperelli suggested that the 57th might fly down to support the ARVN assault. But Stilwell said no. Temperelli handed over the generators and left, taking with him a promise that they would be returned after the operation. Only one ever made it back, and the 57th was totally grounded from 17 November to 15 December. When he recovered the one generator, Temperelli shifted the 57th's one flying aircraft back and forth between Nha Trang and Qui Nhon to provide some coverage at each location.

A graver danger to the 57th's independence developed out of its medical mission. For most of the Korean War, Army ambulance helicopters had served under the aegis of the Army Medical Service, attached to the hospitals behind the corps areas. But in September 1962 General Stilwell considered ending this policy in Vietnam by transferring the 57th from the Medical Service to the Army Transportation Corps, which then controlled all other Army helicopters in Vietnam. Temperelli, accompanied by Lt. Col. Carl A. Fischer, USASGV Surgeon and commander of the 8th Field Hospital, again went to Saigon. This time he was more successful, convincing Stilwell to maintain the old policy.

Temperelli also deflected other attacks on the 57th's integrity. Because of the relatively few hours flown by the pilots in their first year in Vietnam, other Army aviators there argued against dedicating any helicopters to medical evacuation. Some suggested removing the red crosses from medical helicopters and assigning general support tasks to any idle medical aircraft. In another attempt to coopt the 57th's resources, the senior MAAG advisor in Qui Nhon tried several times to commandeer a standby evacuation ship; but each time the 57th told him that he could have priority on the craft only if he were a casualty. All in all, 1962 was not a good year for the air ambulance unit and its pilots.

Early in January 1963, however, an ARVN assault in the Delta convinced many skeptics that the 57th ought to be brought closer to the scene of battle. South Vietnamese intelligence had heard of an enemy radio station operating near the village of Ap Bac in the Plain of Reeds. Fifty U.S. advisers and 400 men of the ARVN 7th Infantry Division flew ten CH–21 Shawnee helicopters to the area. Five armed UH–1's that would serve as close air cover escorted the convoy.

The first three waves of helicopters dropped their troops into the landing zone without difficulty. But just as the fourth wave was touching down, Viet Cong opened fire with automatic weapons and shot down four of the CH–21's. A U.S. Army UH–1B moved into the face of the enemy fire to try to rescue one of the downed crews. It too crashed—the first UH–1B destroyed by the enemy in the Vietnam War. The other four UH–1's suppressed the Viet Cong fire, allowing the remaining Shawnees to leave the hotly contested area without further loss.

Other than for the unusually large number of forces involved, the battle was typical for this period: in the ground fight that followed, the South Vietnamese infantry failed to surround the Viet Cong, who escaped under cover of night. Three American advisers and sixty-five ARVN soldiers were killed. The 57th Medical Detachment, still stationed at Nha Trang and Qui Nhon, far to the north, could not help evacuate the wounded.

The losses suffered at Ap Bac impressed on Army commanders that the air ambulances might be best employed near the fighting. On 16 January the Support Group ordered the 57th to move to Saigon. By this time the 57th had only one flyable aircraft, at Qui Nhon. But Support Group told Captain Temperelli that new UH–1B's were on the way. On 30 January the 57th arrived at Tan Son Nhut Air Base in Saigon.

Dust Off Takes Form

The pilots and crews found Saigon much different from Qui Nhon and Nha Trang. Here they enjoyed access to a large, fully stocked post exchange and commissary. Local Vietnamese stores sold French wines, liqueurs, and champagnes, and the post exchange sold popular American spirits. The Armed Forces Radio Station broadcast the latest American music and reported ball game scores. The officers had clubs in the Brink and Rex Hotels, and the Five Oceans Club in the Cholon Officers' Open Mess. The French-sponsored Cercle Sportif provided the officers swimming and tennis, and the Club Nautique offered water-skiing, rowing, and motorboating. Also available were the Saigon Tennis Club, the Saigon Golf Club, and the Cercle Hippique for horseback riding. The city even boasted a six-lane bowling alley. Some of the pilots frequented cafes like the Riverboat Restaurant, and one even sang for a while in a downtown nightclub.

The veterans had little time to enjoy such amenities. In late February 1963 Captain Temperelli passed the reins of the 57th to a new commander, Maj. Lloyd E. Spencer. The veteran pilots rotated out of Vietnam and their replacements arrived. Shortly after Spencer arrived in Saigon, General Stilwell called him in for an interview. Slapping at a map of South Vietnam, Stilwell asked Spencer how he proposed to cover all the country with only five aircraft. All that Spencer could say was that the 57th would do its best. After a lengthy discussion of problems, Stilwell again promised the 57th the first five new UH–1B's in South Vietnam. On 11 March the unit signed over the last of its grounded UH–1A's for return to the States. The next day Support Group issued the detachment five new UH–1B's that were still on a ship in the Saigon Harbor. On 23 March the 57th declared itself fully operational again.

But Saigon brought its own problems. The 57th's assigned parking area at Tan Son Nhut Airport was directly behind the area where the Vietnamese Air Force pilots parked their C–47 Dakotas. When the VNAF pilots started their planes, always parked with the tails towards the 57th's area, the engines spattered oil all over the bubbles, windows, and windshields of the Hueys. Several times the 57th's crews asked the Vietnamese to park the C-47's facing another direction, but the pilots refused. The 57th's solution to the problem, while it did not foster allied harmony, was effective. Spencer explained: "When you fly a helicopter over the tail of a C-47 it really plays hell with the plane's rear elevators; so the Vietnamese got the message and moved the C-47's."

In April, part of the 57th's pilots and crews bade farewell to the comforts of Saigon when two of the aircraft went on a semipermanent standby to the town of Pleiku, some 120 kilometers northwest of the 57th's old base at Qui Nhon. Pleiku lies in Vietnam's Annamite mountain chain. That month a 57th helicopter at Pleiku joined a search and rescue mission for a B-26 that had crashed while covering a combat assault. The crew found the B-26 lying on a pinnacle, but could not land because of the stunted trees and other growth that covered the peak. While the pilot hovered as low as possible, the crew chief and the medical corpsman leaped from the Huey to the ground, where they cut out a landing area. The Huey landed and the men removed the B-26's .50-caliber machine guns and the bodies of its three Air Force crewmen.

The 57th's two units in the north stood duty round the clock, until their operational commanders canceled night missions after a transport aircraft went down on a flight in darkness over the South China Sea. Most of their missions were to small U.S. Army Special Forces teams scattered among the Montagnard villages in the wild highlands. The Viet Cong there had none of the sophisticated weapons used by their compatriots in the south. The air ambulances at Pleiku contended with only homemade guns, crossbows, and a few firearms the Viet Cong had captured from ARVN troops.

In late June, one of the Hueys at Pleiku moved to Qui Nhon to resume coverage of that sector. In I Corps Zone to the north, U.S. Marine H-34 helicopters furnished both combat aviation support and medical evacuation. The 57th's aircraft at Pleiku and Qui Nhon covered II Corps Zone, and the three in Saigon covered III and IV Corps Zones. Although all the four corps regions of South Vietnam had some form of medical evacuation, it was thinly spread.

For the past year the 57th had worked without a tactical call sign, simply using "Army" and the tail number of the aircraft. For example, if a pilot were flying a helicopter with the serial number 62-12345, his call sign would be "Army 12345." The 57th communicated internally on any vacant frequency it could find. Major Spencer decided that this slapdash system had to go. In Saigon he visited Navy Support Activity, which controlled all the call words in South Vietnam. He received a Signal Operations Instructions book that listed all the unused call words. Most, like "Bandit," were more suitable for assault units than for medical evacuation units. But one entry, "Dust Off," epitomized the 57th's medical evacuation missions. Since the countryside then was dry and dusty, helicopter pickups in the fields often blew dust, dirt, blankets, and shelter halves all over the men on the ground. By adopting "Dust Off," Spencer found for Army aeromedical evacuation in Vietnam a name that lasted the rest of the war.

Even though distinguished by its own name, the 57th still had no formal mission statement. Its pilots worked on the assumption that their main purpose was to evacuate wounded and injured U.S. civilians and military personnel. It continued to provide this service to the Vietnamese as well when resources permitted. Like Captain Temperelli, Major Spencer also felt pressure to allow ground commanders to use Dust Off aircraft for routine administrative flights, but with General Stilwell's support he kept the 57th focused on its medical mission. If the 57th had already scheduled one of its aircraft for a routine flight, it sometimes accepted healthy passengers on a space-available basis, with the proviso that the passengers might have to leave the ship in the middle of nowhere if the pilot received a Dust Off request while in the air.

As the year went on, the 57th flew Dust Off missions more often. On one day alone, 10 September 1963, it evacuated 197 Vietnamese from the Delta, where large Viet Cong forces had virtually destroyed three settlements. That day Dust Off helicopters made flights with Vietnamese jammed into the passenger compartment and standing on the skids. The last flight out took place at night, and the three aircraft flew near a firefight on the ground. After a few tracer rounds arced up toward their helicopters, the pilots blacked out their ships and flew on to Saigon.

The first nine months of the year had brought important changes. Dust Off had a name, solid support from above, a mission—though no mission statement—and a great deal more business. Its problems reflected its new-found popularity.

Relations with the South Vietnamese

Although the number of Vietnamese casualties rose in 1963, the South Vietnamese military refused to set up its own aeromedical evacuation unit. The VNAF response to requests for medical evacuation depended on aircraft availability, the security of the landing zone, and the mood and temperament of the VNAF pilots. If the South Vietnamese had no on-duty or standby aircraft ready to fly a medical evacuation mission they passed the request on to the 57th.

Even when they accepted the mission themselves, their response usually suffered from a lack of leadership and poor organization. Since South Vietnamese air mission commanders rarely flew with their flights, the persons responsible for deciding whether to abort a mission often lacked the requisite experience. As a MACV summary said: "Usually the decision was made to abort, and the air mission commander could do nothing about it. When an aggressive pilot was in the lead ship, the aircraft came through despite the firing. American advisers reported that on two occasions only the first one or two helicopters landed; the rest hovered out of reach of the wounded who needed to get aboard."

An example of the poor quality of VNAF medical evacuation occurred in late October 1963, when the ARVN 2d Battalion, 14th Regiment, conducted Operation LONG HUU II near O Lac in the Delta. At dawn the battalion began its advance. Shortly after they moved out, the Viet Cong ambushed them, opening fire from three sides with automatic weapons and 81-mm. mortars. At 0700 casualty reports started coming into the battalion command post. The battalion commander sent his first casualty report to the regimental headquarters at 0800: one ARVN soldier dead and twelve wounded, with more casualties in the paddies. He then requested medical evacuation helicopters. By 0845 the casualty count had risen to seventeen lightly wounded, fourteen seriously wounded, and four dead. He sent out another urgent call for helicopters. The battalion executive officer and the American adviser prepared two landing zones, one marked by green smoke for the seriously wounded and a second by yellow smoke for the less seriously wounded. Not until 1215 did three VNAF H-34's arrive over O Lac to carry out the wounded and dead. During the delay the ARVN battalion stayed in place to protect their casualties rather than pursue the retreating enemy. The American adviser wrote later: "It is common that, when casualties are sustained, the advance halts while awaiting evacuation. Either the reaction time for helicopter evacuation must be improved, or some plan must be made for troops in the battalion rear to provide security for the evacuation and care of casualties."

The ARVN medical services also proved inadequate to handle the large numbers of casualties. In the Delta, ARVN patients were usually taken to the Vietnamese Provincial Hospital at Can Tho. As the main treatment center for the Delta, it often had a backlog of patients. At night only one doctor was on duty, for the ARVN medical service lacked physicians. If Dust Off flew in a large number of casualties, that doctor normally treated as many as he could; but he rarely called in any of his fellow doctors to help. In return they would not call him on his night off. Many times at night Dust Off pilots would have to make several flights into Can Tho. On return flights the pilots often found loads of injured ARVN soldiers lying on the landing pad where they had been left some hours earlier. After several such flights few pilots could sustain any enthusiasm for night missions.

Another problem was that the ARVN officers sometimes bowed to the sentiments of their soldiers, many of whom believed that the soul lingers between this world and the next if the body is not properly buried. They insisted that Dust Off ships fly out dead bodies, especially if there were no seriously wounded waiting for treatment. Once, after landing at a pickup site north of Saigon, a Dust Off crew saw many ARVN wounded lying on the ground. But the other ARVN soldiers brought bodies to the helicopter to be evacuated first. As the soldiers loaded the dead in one side of the ship, a Dust Off medical corpsman pulled the bodies out the other side. The pilot stepped out of the helicopter to explain in halting French to the ARVN commander that his orders were to carry out only the wounded. But an ARVN soldier manning a .50-caliber machine gun on a nearby armored personnel carrier suddenly pointed his weapon at the Huey. This convinced the Dust Off crew to fly out the bodies. They carried out one load but did not return for another.

Kelly and the Dust Off Mystique

Early in 1964 the growing burden of aeromedical evacuation fell on the 57th's third group of new pilots, crews, and maintenance personnel. The helicopters were still the 1963 UH–1B models, but most of the new pilots were fresh from flight school. The new commander, Maj. Charles L. Kelly, from Georgia, was a gruff, stubborn, dedicated soldier who let few obstacles prevent him from finishing a task. Within six months he set an example of courage and hard work that Dust Off pilots emulated for the rest of the war.

Kelly quickly took advantage of the 57th's belated move to the fighting in the south. On 1 March 1964 Support Group ordered the aircraft at Pleiku and Qui Nhon to move to the Delta. Two helicopters and five pilots, now called Detachment A, 57th Medical Detachment (Helicopter Ambulance), Provisional, flew to the U.S. base at Soc Trang. Once a fighter base for both the French and the Japanese, Soc Trang was a compound roughly 1,000 by 3,000 feet, surrounded by rice paddies.

Unit statistics soon proved the wisdom of the move south: the number of evacuees climbed from 193 in February to 416 in March. Detachment A continued its coverage of combat in the Delta until October 1964, when another helicopter ambulance detachment from the States took over that area. Major Kelly, who had taken command of the 57th on 11 January, moved south with Detachment A, preferring the field and flying to ground duty in Saigon.

Detachment A in Soc Trang lived in crude "Southeast Asia" huts with sandbags and bunkers for protection against enemy mortar and ground attack. The rest of the 57th in Saigon struggled along with air conditioning, private baths, a mess hall, and a bar in their living quarters. In spite of the contrast, most pilots preferred Soc Trang. It was there that Major Kelly and his pilots forged the Dust Off tradition of valorous and dedicated service.

Major Kelly and his teams also benefited from two years of growing American involvement in Vietnam. By the spring of 1964 the United States had 16,000 military personnel in South Vietnam (3,700 officers and 12,300 enlisted men). The Army, which accounted for 10,100 of these, had increased its aircraft in South Vietnam from 40 in December 1961 to 370 in December 1963. For the first time since its arrival two years ago the 57th was receiving enough Dust Off requests to keep all its pilots busy.

But Major Kelly faced one big problem when he arrived: the helicopters that the 57th had received the year before were showing signs of age and use, and General Stilwell, the Support Group commander, could find no new aircraft for the detachment. Average flight time on the old UH–1B's was 800 hours. But this did not deter the new pilots from each flying more than 100 hours a month in medical evacuations. Some of them stopped logging their flight time at 140 hours, so that the flight surgeon would not ground them for exceeding the monthly ceiling.

The new team continued and even stepped up night operations. In April 1963 the detachment flew 110 hours at night while evacuating ninety-nine patients. To aid their night missions in the Delta the pilots made a few special plotting flights, during which they sketched charts of the possible landing zones, outlined any readily identifiable terrain features, and noted whether radio navigational aid could be received.

During one such flight Major Kelly and his copilot heard on their radio that a VNAF T–28, a fixed-wing plane, had gone down. After joining the search, Kelly soon located the plane. While he and his crew circled the area trying to decide how to approach the landing zone, the Viet Cong below opened fire on the helicopter. One round passed up through the open cargo door and slammed into the ceiling. Unfazed, Kelly shot a landing to the T–28, taking fire from all sides. Once down, he, his crew chief, and his medical corpsman jumped out and sprayed submachine gun fire at the Viet Cong while helping the VNAF pilot destroy his radios and pull the M60 machine guns from his plane. Kelly left the area without further damage and returned the VNAF pilot to his unit. Kelly and his Dust Off crew flew more than 500 miles that day.

On 2 April one of the Detachment A crews flying to Saigon from Soc Trang received a radio call that a village northwest of them had been overrun. Flying up to the area where the Mekong River flows into South Vietnam from Cambodia, they landed at the village of Cai Cai, where during the night Viet Cong had killed or wounded all the people. Soldiers lay at their battle stations where they had fallen, women and children where they had been shot. The Dust Off teams worked the rest of the day flying out the dead and wounded, putting two or three children on each litter.

One night that spring Detachment A pilots Capt. Patrick H. Brady and 2d Lt. Ernest J. Sylvester were on duty when a call came in that an A1–E Skyraider, a fixed-wing plane, had gone down near the town of Rach Gia. Flying west to the site, they radioed the Air Force radar controller, who guided them to the landing zone and warned them of Viet Cong antiaircraft guns. As the Dust Off ship drew near the landing zone, which was plainly marked by the burning A1–E, the pilot of another nearby A1–E radioed that he had already knocked out the Viet Cong machine guns. But when Brady and Sylvester approached the zone the Viet Cong opened fire. Bullets crashed into the cockpit and the pilots lost control of the aircraft. Neither was seriously wounded and they managed to regain control and hurry out of the area. Viet Cong fire then brought down the second A1–E. A third arrived shortly and finally suppressed the enemy fire, allowing a second Dust Off ship from Soc Trang to land in the zone. The crew chief and medical corpsman found what they guessed was the dead pilot of the downed aircraft, then found the pilot of the second, who had bailed out, and flew him back to Soc Trang.

A short time later Brady accompanied an ARVN combat assault mission near Phan Thiet, northeast of Saigon. While Brady's Dust Off ship circled out of range of enemy ground fire, the transport helicopters landed and the troops moved out into a wooded area heavily defended by the Viet Cong. The ARVN soldiers immediately suffered several casualties and called for Dust Off. Brady's aircraft took hits going into and leaving the landing zone, but he managed to fly out the wounded. In Phan Thiet, while he was assessing the damage to his aircraft, an American adviser asked him if he would take ammunition back to the embattled ARVN unit when he returned for the next load of wounded. After discussing the propriety of carrying ammunition in an aircraft marked with red crosses, Brady and his pilots decided to consider the ammunition as "preventive medicine" and fly it in to the ARVN troops. Back at the landing zone Brady found that Viet Cong fire had downed an L–19 observation plane. Brady ran to the crash site but both the American pilot and the observer had been killed. The medical corpsman and crew chief pulled the bodies from the wreckage and loaded them on the helicopter. Brady left the ammunition and flew out with the dead.

By the time the helicopter had finished its mission and returned to

Tan Son Nhut, most of the 57th were waiting. News of an American death traveled quickly in those early days of the war. Later, reflecting on the incident, Kelly praised his pilots for bringing the bodies back even though the 57th's mission statement said nothing about moving the dead. But he voiced renewed doubts about the ferrying of ammunition.

In fact, the Dust Off mission was again under attack. When Support Command began to pressure the 57th to place removable red crosses on the aircraft and begin accepting general purpose missions, Kelly stepped up unit operations. Knowing that removable red crosses had already been placed on transport and assault helicopters in the north, Kelly told his men that the 57th must prove its worth— and by implication the value of dedicated medical helicopters—beyond any shadow of doubt.

Whereas the 57th before had flown missions only in response to a request, it now began to seek missions. Kelly himself flew almost every night. As dusk came, he and his crew would depart Soc Trang and head southwest for the marshes and Bac Lieu, home of a team from the 73d Aviation Company and detachments from two signal units, then further south to Ca Mau, an old haunt of the Viet Minh, whom the French had never been able to dislodge from its forested swamps. Next they would fly south almost to the tip of Ca Mau Peninsula, then at Nam Can reverse their course toward the Seven Canals area. After a check for casualties there at Vi Thanh, they turned northwest up to Rach Gia on the Gulf of Siam, then on to the Seven Mountains region on the Cambodian border. From there they came back to Can Tho, the home of fourteen small American units, then up to Vinh Long on the Mekong River, home of the 114th Airmobile Company. Next they flew due east to Truc Giang, south to the few American advisers at Phu Vinh, then home to Soc Trang. The entire circuit was 720 kilometers.

If any of the stops had patients to be evacuated, Kelly's crew loaded them on the aircraft and continued on course, unless a patient's condition warranted returning immediately to Soc Trang. After delivering the patients, they would sometimes resume the circuit. Many nights they carried ten to fifteen patients who otherwise would have had to wait until daylight to receive the care they needed. In March this flying from outpost to outpost, known as "scarfing," resulted in seventy-four hours of night flying that evacuated nearly one-fourth of that month's 450 evacuees. The strategem worked; General Stilwell dropped the idea of having the 57th use removable red crosses.

Although most of Dust Off's work in the Delta was over flat, marshy land, Detachment A sometimes had to work the difficult mountainous areas near the Cambodian border. Late on the afternoon of 11 April Kelly received a mission request to evacuate two wounded ARVN soldiers from Phnom Kto Mountain of the Seven Mountains of An Giang Province. When he arrived he found that the only landing zone near the ground troops was a small area surrounded by high trees below some higher ground held by the Viet Cong. Despite the updrafts common to mountain flying, the mists, and the approaching darkness, Kelly shot an approach to the area. The enemy opened fire and kept firing until Kelly's ship dropped below the treetops into the landing zone. Kelly could set the aircraft down on only one skid; the slope was too steep. Since only one of the wounded was at the landing zone, Kelly and his crew had to balance the ship precariously while waiting for the ARVN troops to carry the other casualty up the mountain. With both patients finally on board, Kelly took off and again flew through enemy fire. The medical corpsman promptly began working on the Vietnamese, one of whom had been wounded in five places. Both casualties survived.

When Kelly flew such a mission he rarely let bad weather, darkness, or the enemy stop him from completing it. He fought his way to the casualties and brought them out. On one mission the enemy forced him away from the landing zone before he could place the patients on board. An hour later he tried to land exactly the same way, through enemy fire, and this time he managed to load the patients safely. The Viet Cong showed their indifference to the red crosses on the aircraft by trying to destroy it with small arms, automatic weapons, and mortars, even while the medical corpsman and crew chief loaded the patients. One round hit the main fuel drain valve and JP–4 fuel started spewing. Kelly elected to fly out anyway, practicing what he had preached since he arrived in Vietnam by putting the patients above all else and hurrying them off the battlefield. He radioed the Soc Trang tower that his ship was leaking fuel and did not have much left, and that he wanted priority on landing. The tower operator answered that Kelly had priority and asked whether he needed anything else. Kelly said, "Yes, bring me some ice cream." Just after he landed on the runway the engine quit, fuel tanks empty. Crash trucks surrounded the helicopter. The base commander drove up, walked over to Kelly, and handed him a quart of ice cream.

Apart from the Viet Cong, the 57th's greatest problem at that time was a lack of pilots. After Kelly reached Vietnam he succeeded in having the other nine Medical Service Corps pilots who followed him assigned to the 57th. He needed more, but the Surgeon General's Aviation Branch seemed to have little understanding of the rigors of Dust Off flying. In the spring of 1964 the Aviation Branch tried to have new Medical Service Corps pilots assigned to nonmedical helicopter units in Vietnam, assuming that they would benefit more from combat training than from Dust Off flying. In late June Kelly gave his response:

As for combat experience, the pilots in this unit are getting as much or more combat-support flying experience than any unit over here. You must understand that everybody wants to get into the Aeromedical Evacuation Business. To send pilots to U.T.T. [a nonmedical unit] or anywhere else is playing right into their hands. I fully realize that I do not know much about the big program, but our job is evacuation of casualties from the battlefield. This we are doing day and night, without escort aircraft, and with only one ship for each mission. The other [nonmedical] units fly in groups, rarely at night, and always heavily armed.

In other words, Kelly thought that his unit had a unique job to do and that the only effective training for it could be found in the cockpit of a Dust Off helicopter.

With more and more fighting occurring in the Delta and around Saigon, the 57th could not always honor every evacuation request. U.S. Army helicopter assault companies were forced to keep some of their aircraft on evacuation standby, but without a medical corpsman or medical equipment. Because of the shortage of Army aviators and the priority of armed combat support, the Medical Service Corps did not have enough pilots to staff another Dust Off unit in Vietnam. Most Army aeromedical evacuation units elsewhere already worked with less than their permitted number of pilots. Although Army aviation in Vietnam had grown considerably since 1961, by the summer of 1964 its resources fell short of what it needed to perform its missions, especially medical evacuation.

Army commanders, however, seldom have all the men and material they can use, and Major Kelly knew that he had to do his best with what he had. On the morning of 1 July 1964 Kelly received a mission request from an ARVN unit in combat near Vinh Long. An American sergeant, the adviser, had been hit in the leg by shrapnel from a mortar round. Several of the ARVN infantry were also wounded. Kelly and his crew flew to the area. The Viet Cong were close in to the ARVN soldiers and the fighting continued as Kelly's helicopter came in to a hover. Kelly floated his ship back and forth, trying to spot the casualties. The Viet Cong opened fire on his ship. The ARVN soldiers and their American advisers were staying low. One adviser radioed Kelly to get out of the area. He answered, "When I have your wounded." Many rounds hit his aircraft before one of them passed through the open side door and pierced his heart. He murmured "My God," and died. His ship pitched up, nosed to the right, rolled over, and crashed.

The rest of the crew, shaken but not seriously injured, crawled from the wreck and dragged Kelly's body behind a mound of dirt. Dust Off aircraft later evacuated Kelly's crew and the other casualties.

The United States awarded him the Distinguished Service Cross posthumously. South Vietnam conferred the Military Order Medal of Vietnam, National Order, Fifth Class, and the Cross of Gallantry with Palm. Far more important than the medals he earned was his legacy to the hundreds of Dust Off pilots who followed him. His death saddened all who had known him, for he had given so much of himself so selflessly. The men of the 57th heard that General Stilwell, Kelly's commander for the last six months, wept when he heard of his death.

Capt. Paul A. Bloomquist took command of the 57th Medical Detachment in Saigon and Capt. Patrick H. Brady moved to Soc Trang to take over Detachment A. Assuming that the 57th would now select its missions more carefully, the commander of the 13th Aviation Battalion in the Delta called Brady into his office. He asked what changes would be made now that Kelly was gone. Brady told him that the 57th would continue flying missions exactly as Kelly had taught them, accepting any call for help.

A New Buildup

Kelly's death coincided with an important turning point in U.S. relations with North and South Vietnam. In the first half of 1964 the new administration of President Lyndon B. Johnson concluded that the growing political and military disturbances in South Vietnam required a commitment of larger U.S. economic and military resources in the area. In March 1964, after visiting South Vietnam, Secretary of Defense Robert McNamara recommended that the United States increase its aid to the Republic of Vietnam. President Johnson immediately increased U.S. aid to South Vietnam by $60 million. He also promised to obtain new equipment for the South Vietnamese Army, to finance a 50,000-man increase in South Vietnamese forces, and to provide funds for the modernization of the country's government. At his request the Joint Chiefs of Staff began to draft plans for the retaliatory bombing of North Vietnam. Over the next few months the South Vietnamese government of Maj. Gen. Nguyen Khanh was unable to make good use of the increased U.S. aid; American advisers in the countryside reported that Khanh's political power was still crumbling. General Khanh and Air Commodore Nguyen Cao Ky, commander of the South Vietnamese Air Force, began a public campaign to place all blame for the deteriorating conditions on North Vietnam and draw the United States even further into the conflict.

The United States was already more deeply involved than most Americans knew. For some time United States forces had taken part in clandestine amphibious raids on the North Vietnamese coast to gather intelligence. In the spring of 1964 the Johnson administration publicly stated that the United States was stockpiling for the possible deployment of large numbers of American troops in Southeast Asia

The administration also surrounded with great publicity the dedication of the new U.S.-built airbase at Da Nang, on the northernmost part of South Vietnam's coast.

These American threats had no effect on the Viet Cong or the North Vietnamese, who continued to bring supplies south through trails in Laos and to stage daring terrorist raids even in the center of Saigon. The North Vietnamese Navy openly challenged the United States in early August 1964 when its torpedo patrol boats attacked two U.S. destroyers sailing in the Gulf of Tonkin. Congress, outraged by this seemingly unprovoked attack in international waters, quickly gave President Johnson nearly unanimous approval to take whatever measures he thought necessary to protect U.S. forces in the area.

As U.S. involvement mounted, the requests made by Kelly and Stilwell for another air ambulance unit at last took effect. In August the Surgeon General's Office named five more helicopter ambulance detachments for assignment to Southeast Asia. The 82d Medical Detachment (Helicopter Ambulance) at Fort Sam Houston, Texas, was alerted for a 1 October move. The other four detachments were put on notice without firm departure dates and told to bring their units to full strength.

The advance party of the 82d arrived in Saigon on 5 October, and the next day Support Group, Vietnam, gave the detachment five new UH–1B's. The rest of the detachment arrived two weeks later. The officers and enlisted men of the 82d spent their first nights in Saigon billeted with their counterparts in the 57th. There they heard disturbing war stories from the veterans, then left for their new home in Soc Trang. Most of the detachment traveled by convoy, down Route 4 through the alien Delta countryside. Their first sight of Soc Trang — a small airstrip with a tiny village at one end, lying in the middle of rice paddies, with only a triple-stranded concertina wire to protect the perimeter — added to their concern.

To stagger personnel departure dates and help train the new 82d pilots and crews in Dust Off flying, three of the 57th pilots transferred to the 82d, and three from the 82d transferred to the 57th. Maj. Henry P. Capozzi commanded the 82d; Maj. Howard H. Huntsman, the 57th. The 82d used the 57th's Hueys until it had its own in place and declared itself operational on 7 November 1964.

The new unit retraced the steps of their predecessors. Soon after they started flying evacuation missions the pilots of the 82d had their first taste of Viet Cong resistance. On a mission near Bac Lieu on 27 October, one of their new helicopters took three hits during a takeoff with casualties aboard. The crew flew back to Soc Trang and found one bullet hole through the red cross on one of the cargo doors. One of the ARVN evacuees lay dead from an enemy round that had penetrated the aircraft.

The old question of a call sign soon came up. After considering various signs, including those used by helicopter ambulance units in Korea, the new commanders settled on the 57th's sign, "Dust Off." When the 82d also adopted the 57th's unit emblem, merely changing the "57th" to "82d," some of the former 57th pilots objected to this piracy. But the policy made sense, since both units performed the same mission and the common symbols helped the ground forces recognize the ambulance helicopters.

One radical change was the conservative style of Capozzi and Huntsman. Both felt that the "wild and wooly days" ought to end and that the pilots of the 57th and 82d ought to temper their flying with cool judgment. They counseled their pilots to accept no missions without direct communication with the ground forces requesting the mission, to fly night missions only for extreme emergencies, and never to fly into an insecure landing zone. Despite these orders, the veterans of the 57th at Soc Trang quietly instilled the old élan in the new pilots, ensuring that the Kelly spirit stayed with Dust Off until the end of the war.

In one area, however, Capozzi and Huntsman succeeded in ending a Kelly practice. They refused to allow their pilots to fly the Delta looking for patients. "Shopping for business," they said, "is a waste of time." They reasoned that the communication net was now secure enough to ensure speedy response to any call. The decision was sound. With five new helicopters, Dust Off no longer had to cover 31,000 square kilometers with only two flyable aircraft. U.S. advisers could call or relay their mission requests directly to the air ambulance units via FM radio; ARVN units in the Delta routed their calls through the joint U.S.-ARVN Combat Operations Center at the 13th Aviation Battalion (U.S.). The aircraft pilots decided on missions. Air Force radar control at Can Tho provided its customary invaluable service; the rapport of USAF radar controllers with pilots of the 82d was as excellent as it was with those of the 57th.

In other respects, Kelly's teachings lived. As casualties mounted in the first months of 1965, the pilots of the 82d, despite their commander's caution, flew many night missions. Since the Viet Cong usually attacked outposts and villages at night, and both sides patrolled and set ambushes at night, the Dust Off pilots too had to be abroad, seeking the wounded where they lay.

The Crisis Deepens

Late in 1964, the *271st* and *272d Viet Cong Regiments* merged and equipped themselves with new Chinese and Soviet weapons, forming the *9th Viet Cong Division*. The *9th Division* showed the value of this change in a battle for Binh Gia, a small Catholic village on Inter provincial Route 2, sixty-five kilometers southeast of Saigon. On 28 December and over the next three days the Viet Cong ambushed and nearly destroyed the South Vietnamese 33d Ranger Battalion and 4th Marine Battalion, and inflicted heavy casualties on the armored and mechanized forces that came to their rescue. The reorganized and reequipped Viet Cong were so confident that they stood and fought a four-day pitched battle rather than employ their usual hit-and-run tactics. The South Vietnamese suffered over 400 casualties and lost more than 200 weapons. Nearly eighty helicopters, including those from the 57th Medical Detachment, took part in the relief operations of this battle. During the fighting, Dust Off rescued nine crewmen from their downed helicopters and evacuated scores of South Vietnamese troops.

Assistant Secretary of State William P. Bundy urged President Johnson to retaliate against North Vietnam. He was seconded by the new commander of the Military Assistance Command in Vietnam, Gen. William C. Westmoreland, and the U.S. ambassador to South Vietnam, Gen. Maxwell D. Taylor. Westmoreland thought that the Viet Cong seemed to be preparing to move from guerrilla tactics to a more conventional war. But President Johnson, ignoring his advisers, refused to allow an immediate bombing campaign against North Vietnam.

Shortly afterward, however, Johnson himself lost confidence in current U.S. and South Vietnamese policy. On the morning of 7 February the Viet Cong attacked the U.S. advisers' base and airstrip at Camp Holloway near Pleiku. Mortar fire and demolitions killed several Americans, wounded more than a hundred, and destroyed five aircraft. Within hours forty-nine U.S. Navy fighter-bombers struck back at a North Vietnamese barracks just above the Demilitarized Zone. In his memoirs General Westmoreland called this strike a vital juncture in the history of American involvement in Southeast Asia. Within two days President Johnson approved a policy of "sustained reprisal" against the North.

Along with the rest of the U.S. Army in Vietnam, Dust Off quickly felt the new surge of America's war effort. From 1962 to early 1965 the Dust Off pilots and their crewmen had been at school in Vietnam. Now they would have to show what they had learned, applying on a large scale the tradition of courage and unhesitating service that they had forged in the early years.

CHAPTER III

The System Matures

Early in 1965 a growing number of Viet Cong attacks on U.S. personnel in South Vietnam prompted President Johnson to order all American dependents out of that country. On 22 February General Westmoreland asked for American combat ground forces to defend allied bases against Viet Cong attacks, and on 25 February Secretary of State Dean Rusk approved. On 8 March the first of these forces, a battalion landing team of the 9th Marine Expeditionary Brigade, debarked on the beaches at Da Nang. U.S. officials announced that the new troops would make several key bases more secure, thereby freeing the South Vietnamese forces to press the war more vigorously. But the Viet Cong continued their terrorist campaign. On 30 March they detonated a powerful bomb outside the hotel housing the U.S. Embassy in Saigon. The explosion killed twenty-one people, including two Americans, and wounded two hundred others, including fifty-two Americans.

After a lull in the fighting while the Viet Cong waited out the dry season, which favored the superior mobility of the ARVN forces, the countryside erupted in May. A Viet Cong regiment attacked Song Be, the capital of Phuoc Long province in northern III Corps Zone. Soon a more serious blow came when the rebels ambushed an ARVN battalion and destroyed the column sent to its aid. In June the enemy again dealt the ARVN forces a heavy blow at Dong Xoai, ninety-six kilometers northeast of Saigon. June also brought the collapse of the current South Vietnamese governing coalition, and the new rulers, Generals Nguyen Van Thieu and Nguyen Cao Ky, seemed to have little chance of ending the recent years of political instability. In July the fighting shifted to the Central Highlands of II Corps Zone, where the South Vietnamese suffered a series of defeats.

This military and political deterioration in 1965 produced a rapid increase in U.S. aid to South Vietnam. Within a few months of their arrival in March, the first U.S. combat units in South Vietnam began search-and-destroy operations against the Viet Cong near U.S. bases. By the end of the year evidence of increased North Vietnamese infiltration of the South helped General Westmoreland to obtain substantial reinforcements of U.S. combat troops. A U.S. troop buildup continued steadily until March 1968 as the United States expanded its effort to destroy the political and military influence of the National Liberation Front.

Origins of the Air Ambulance Platoon

As more soldiers arrived, the Army Medical Service began its own buildup, which included an increase in the number of medical evacuation units. During the next three years the Surgeon General of the Army sent two air ambulance companies and six more helicopter ambulance companies to Vietnam. In March 1966 the 44th Medical Brigade, which had been activated in January, assumed control of most Army medical units in Vietnam. Over the next two years the brigade began to coordinate the work of the 68th Medical Group (responsible for III and IV Corps Zones), the 43d Group (South II Corps Zone), the 55th Group (North II Corps Zone), and the 67th Group (I Corps Zone). These medical groups, with the exception of the 55th, which left aeromedical evacuation in its area to the 43d Group, commanded all the nondivisional air ambulances — the companies and detachments. In late 1965, with the Surgeon General's permission, American combat forces also brought in Medical Service Corps pilots to man the aircraft of a new form of medical evacuation unit: the air ambulance platoon. Unlike the air ambulance units of the 44th Brigade, it would depend on its combat assault division for command and supply.

The platoon owed its existence to the creation of the first airmobile division in the U.S. Army, the 1st Cavalry Division (Airmobile). In August 1962 the U.S. Army Tactical Mobility Requirements Board, chaired by Lt. Gen. Hamilton H. Howze, had recommended the creation of a new airmobile division, which would be served by an air ambulance platoon. Outlining the probable nature of airmobile warfare the Board had assumed that

...all categories of patients within the theater of operations will be evacuated by air. AMEDS aircraft organic to the division will evacuate casualties from forward pickup sites and/or aid stations to clearing stations or Mobile Army Surgical Hospitals. Air Ambulance companies assigned to corps and field Army will evacuate casualties from the clearing stations and surgical hospitals to evacuation hospitals.

Although the air ambulance battalion would use several types of helicopters, the air ambulance platoon would usually consist of only twelve UH–1's.

In early 1963 the Army decided to test the precepts laid out by the Howze Board. On 7 January the Deputy Chief of Staff for Operations issued instructions for the creation of an experimental air assault division. The unit was organized in February at Fort Benning, Georgia, and named the 11th Air Assault Division (Test). Its commander was Brig. Gen. Harry W. O. Kinnard.

The division was composed of eight infantry battalions (expanded to nine in Vietnam) organized into three brigades: three battalions each for the 1st and 2d Brigades and two for the 3d Brigade. One brigade had an airborne capability. An artillery battalion in each brigade provided ground-to-ground fire support and an Aerial Rocket Artillery Battery provided air-to-ground support. The thirty-six UH–1B's of the aerial rocket battery each carried seventy-two folding fin rockets, and most also carried externally-mounted M60 machine guns. An aviation battery of sixteen light observation helicopters coordinated the division's artillery. Two assault helicopter battalions each had sixty unarmed helicopters, organized into three companies of twenty ships each. Both battalions had an armed helicopter company of twelve UH–1B gunships, each carrying four M60's and fifteen rockets. As the Howze Board had suggested, the Air Ambulance Platoon, a structurally new aeromedical evacuation unit, fell under the division's medical battalion.

Air Assault I, a field exercise held at Fort Stewart, Georgia, in September and October 1963, tested the control capabilities of the air assault battalion and company, and the problems of the air ambulance platoon. This exercise and others held at Forts Benning and Gordon suggested that the platoon could effectively support the Air Assault Division without the benefits of a superior company command. Faulty communications equipment and the limited capacity of the UH–1B's were the only serious problems affecting the platoon's performance.

The experimental 11th Air Assault Division was disbanded soon after the testing in Georgia, but its components and the resources of the 2d Infantry Division at Fort Benning were combined and given the name of the 1st Cavalry Division, which had been on duty in Korea since 1950. The new division, the 1st Cavalry Division (Airmobile), had roughly 16,000 men, the standard allotment. But it had 4 1/2 times the standard number of aircraft and one-half the standard number of ground vehicles. It acquired almost one thousand aviators and two thousand aviation mechanics. The creation of this division opened a new phase in U.S. Army warfare.

The Air Ambulance Platoon, which consisted of twelve helicopters and their crews, was an integral part of the new division, and deployed with it to the mountainous Central Highlands of South Vietnam in August 1965. It served as part of the division's 15th Medical Battalion. It not only offered medical evacuation to wounded soldiers of the 1st Cavalry but also had the equipment to rescue pilots of crashed and burning aircraft. It consisted of a medical evacuation section of eight helicopters and a crash rescue section of four helicopters. It also had three Kaman "Sputnik" fire suppression systems to enable the crash rescue teams to enter burning aircraft. Unfortunately, if the aircraft fitted with the Sputnik system also carried its full complement of two firemen, a crew chief, a medical corpsman, and two pilots, it could not lift off unless the crew had drained the fuel tanks to 400 pounds or less. After its arrival in Vietnam the platoon found that maintenance problems, general aircraft shortages, and regular evacuation missions made it impossible to keep four of its aircraft ready at all times for crash rescue missions.

Unlike the helicopter detachments and companies of the 44th Medical Brigade, the platoon's pilots used "Medevac" as their call sign. However, they resembled the pilots of the older units in their methods, training, and outlook. Like the commissioned Dust Off pilots, the platoon's officer pilots had graduated from the helicopter program of the U.S. Army Aviation School at Fort Rucker, Alabama, and had been trained in emergency resuscitative medicine by the Army Medical Department.

The Air Ambulance Platoon Goes to Work

After the 1st Cavalry began to dig in on the An Khe plain in early September 1965 the platoon's pilots flew their first missions and quickly tasted some Viet Cong resistance. To protect the platoon's aircraft, the division began keeping gunships on call for escort. The platoon's pilots, however, thought that traveling with the slower, heavier gunships wasted precious minutes of response time.

During the next three years, a period of large search-and-destroy operations, medical aircraft often accompanied ARVN and U.S. forces to the battlefield. In the remote Central Highlands the 1st Cavalry's air ambulance platoon found it wise to conform to the Howze Board report by evacuating its patients only as far as the battalion aid stations or division clearing stations. Nonorganic air ambulances commanded by medical authorities would then backhaul the casualties to the 71st Evacuation Hospital at Pleiku or to hospitals further away, on the coast. Later in the war, when the 1st Cavalry moved to III Corps Zone, the platoon itself began to make evacuation flights from the site of wounding directly to hospitals.

In time the platoon would prove its value, but some of its early experiences were not encouraging. On 19 September four of the platoon's ships supported an early 1st Cavalry operation. Because of poor coordination and misplaced concern on the part of ground personnel, the transport helicopters carried out the casualties and the air ambulances carried out the dead.

On 10 October one of the platoon's pilots, Capt. Guy Kimsey, answered an evacuation request from a ground unit sixty kilometers east of An Khe. While Kimsey loaded his ship, a Viet Cong round hit the engine and shut down the aircraft. Another helicopter flew the crew and patients back to An Khe, where Kimsey told the 15th Transportation Battalion that he had a downed ship. The maintenance unit sent out an aircraft recovery team the same day, but the team could not find the ship and accused the pilot of giving them the wrong coordinates. Rankled, Kimsey climbed into the recovery aircraft and flew the team chief on the spot. At first, as they approached the area at some distance, Kimsey thought the chief might be right. But as he drew nearer he saw the outline of a helicopter on the ground. They landed. All that he could find of his ship was part of the tail rotor. He checked with the ground troops in the area who had called in the evacuation request. From them he learned that when the Viet Cong had earlier tried to overrun the position, the U.S. troops had called in friendly artillery. One of the rounds had scored a direct hit on the disabled helicopter.

Misfortune struck again on 10 October during Operation SHINY BAYONET near An Khe. Three of the platoon's ships flew out to evacuate eleven seriously wounded soldiers from the 3d Brigade. As they approached the landing zone at 1630, they saw the fires from Air Force tactical strikes still burning. A firefight also raged, and the ground commander radioed that the landing zone was insecure. The senior pilot elected to stay at high altitude with his Huey gunship escort and one other Medevac ship while the third ship made a low approach to the pickup zone. As he took his aircraft in, the pilot of the third ship, Capt. Charles F. Kane, Jr., was struck in the head by an enemy bullet. His copilot flew the aircraft to the 85th Evacuation Hospital, where Kane became the platoon's first fatality.

By mid-October the North Vietnamese Army had begun its drive against allied forces in the Central Highlands. In supporting the ARVN forces that tried to repulse this attack, the 1st Cavalry and its Air Ambulance Platoon received their first severe test. By early October the *32d* and *33d North Vietnamese Regiments* had infiltrated western Pleiku Province between the Cambodian border and Plei Me, a Special Forces base camp forty-three kilometers south of Pleiku. Route 6C stretched north from Plei Me toward Pleiku. A third unit, the *66th North Vietnamese Regiment,* was soon to arrive.

On 20 October the *33d North Vietnamese Regiment* attacked four South Vietnamese Civilian Irregular Defense Group (CIDG) companies at Plei Me. The North Vietnamese *32d Regiment* lay in ambush for the ARVN forces expected to move south from Pleiku. On 23 October the ARVN armored relief force left Pleiku and marched south toward Plei Me, covered by the artillery of the 1st Cavalry Division. On the afternoon of the 24th, Air Ambulance Platoon helicopters carried an artillery liaison party into the column and returned with some noncombat-injured soldiers. At 1750 the Communist ambush struck the convoy, but the ARVN troops broke out and reached the beseiged camp the following day.

Over the next month the 1st Cavalry Division and ARVN forces continued to fight over this territory in the battle of the Ia Drang Valley. On 27 October General Westmoreland ordered Maj. Gen. Harry W.O. Kinnard, 1st Cavalry Division commander, to conduct search-and-destroy operations in western Pleiku Province. For the first time the division's mission was unlimited offense.

In this battle the Air Ambulance Platoon proved its worth. Early in November Lt. Col. Harold G. Moore took his cavalry battalion by helicopter into a landing zone near the Cambodian border. The newly-arrived *66th Regiment* and the remnants of the *33d Regiment* waited on a mountain overlooking the landing zone. Heavy enemy fire from these regiments restricted helicopter approaches and departures, and friendly casualties began to mount. The battalion surgeon, with medical supplies and four medical corpsmen, flew in under heavy enemy fire on an Air Ambulance Platoon ship and immediately began treating the casualties. This saved the lives of many soldiers who could not have survived a long wait for evacuation. By that night the Air Ambulance Platoon and returning gunships had evacuated all the wounded. Although the gunships had helped, the brunt of the evacuation burden had fallen on the Air Ambulance Platoon, which had performed superbly.

At the start of the Ia Drang campaign the Air Ambulance Platoon operated twelve aircraft. One was destroyed on 10 October 1965, four were usually down for maintenance, two were required for division base coverage at An Khe, and two supported the operations of the Republic of Korea (ROK) forces east of An Khe. To support the nearly three thousand men of a reinforced brigade, which was the average strength committed at any one time to the Ia Drang, the 15th Medical Battalion now had only three aircraft to site forward. The casualties varied, but averaged 70 to 80 a day, with 280 on the worst day. Fortunately the troop ships carried the less critically injured men from the landing zones, easing the platoon's load.

In his after-action report, Colonel Moore described another problem he had met in his medical evacuation: the heavy enemy fire and the dense 100-foot high trees had prevented the platoon from evacuating men from the spot where they were wounded. The ground troops had had to move many of the wounded to a single secure landing zone. Moore reported: "I lost many leaders killed and wounded while recovering casualties. Wounded must be pulled back to some type of covered position and then treated. Troops must not get so concerned with casualties that they forget the enemy and their mission. Attempting to carry a man requires up to four men as bearers which can hurt a unit at a critical time." The solution, which came later, involved a technical innovation rather than restraining the soldier's natural concern for his wounded comrades.

By mid-November the 15th Medical Battalion and its Air Ambulance Platoon were short five pilots and fifty-six enlisted men. Of the twelve Medical Service Corps pilots authorized the platoon, one was dead, one was injured, and the battalion commander had placed two on his staff and had reassigned another who had only four months remaining in his tour of duty. The commander asked for replacements, but none could be found because all units were short of men.

Saturday, 18 December, was another dark day for the Air Ambulance Platoon. Capt. Walter L. Berry, Jr., pilot, and WO1 George W. Rice, copilot, had just settled to the ground at a pickup site to evacuate two 1st Cavalry wounded when an enemy soldier opened fire on the helicopter from the left. One bullet, entering through the open cargo door, struck Rice in the head. Another hit the crew chief in the hand. Berry raced to the nearest clearing station, but Rice died there within an hour, the first warrant officer in the Medical Service Corps Aviation Program to be killed in action. The Medevac ship had been unescorted and unarmed. Shortly thereafter the platoon commander, Maj. Carl J. Bobay, wrote: "Within three months of operations in Vietnam, two pilots have been killed, one enlisted man wounded, and nine helicopters shot up, all due to enemy action. Believe me...we are not proud of these statistics. What the next eight months may hold in store for us is too much to even consider."

During this period more of the regular medical detachments were deploying in the two southern Corps Zones. The 283d Medical Detachment (Helicopter Ambulance), activated at Fort Lewis, Washington, landed at Saigon on 1 September 1965 and started to help the 57th cover III Corps Zone. In November 1965, the 254th Medical Detachment (Helicopter Ambulance) also arrived at Tan Son Nhut Airport, Saigon. The two ships that had sailed from Tacoma, Washington, with all the 254th's equipment, reached the South Vietnamese coast on 29 October but could not be unloaded until mid-January because of the congestion in the ports. Until then some of the 254th's pilots worked with the 283d and 57th. The 254th declared itself operational on 1 February at Long Binh with the primary mission of direct support for the 173d Airborne Brigade on its sweep operations in III Corps Zone. The 57th and 283d supported the other allied units in the sector.

The Medical Company (Air Ambulance)

In September 1965 another new type of medical evacuation unit deployed in Vietnam—the medical company (air ambulance). The 1959 table of standard equipment for such a unit provided for twenty-four two-patient helicopters, served by twenty-eight officers and a larger group of enlisted men. In September 1964 the 498th Medical Company (Air Ambulance) was activated at Fort Sam Houston, Texas, where it served in a standby utility capacity until June 1965. That month the company received twenty-five new UH–1D's fresh from the Bell Helicopter Plant, and the pilots set to work learning the new machine.

At Camp Bullis, a subpost of Fort Sam Houston nineteen miles northwest of San Antonio, the company conducted instrument training and practiced the tactics of day and night flying. On most days the flight crews and their instructors took off at 0600 and were still out flying at 2100. All crew members also had some target practice with the M14 rifle and the .45-caliber pistol. Crew chiefs and medical corpsmen practiced firing from the open cargo doors of an airborne helicopter. Most of the flight practice simulated the low-level navigation and approaches that the instructors had learned flying over the Delta in South Vietnam. Because of the varied military occupational specialties of the enlisted men, Lt. Col. Joseph P. Madrano, commander of the 498th, convinced Maj. Gen. William Harris, the post commander, to let the 498th tailor its own unit training program. General Harris not only agreed but also had his staff prepare training aids, and he himself visited the unit almost daily to see if he could do more to help.

On 24 July 1965 a Department of Army message arrived assigning the 498th to U.S. Army, Pacific, destination unstated. Last minute efforts to obtain and pack supplies, aided greatly by General Harris, drew to a close. The 498th planned a well-deserved party for the men and their families at Salado Creek Park in Fort Sam Houston. General Harris, whom they invited, first suggested then insisted that the unit find a civilian UH–1. He wanted the families to have at least one flight in a Huey to see the aircraft that their fathers, sons, and husbands flew. The Bell Helicopter Corporation cooperated and everyone got to ride in a helicopter.

Shortly after he flew into Nha Trang with the advance party of the 498th, Colonel Madrano went to Saigon where the Surgeon of the U.S. Army, Vietnam (USARV) told him that the company would cover the entire II Corps Zone from a base or bases of Madrano's choosing. In the early fall of 1965 the only American combat unit in II Corps Zone was the 1st Brigade of the 101st Airborne Division (Airmobile), which usually operated north of Qui Nhon. Several Special Forces camps monitored the border and a few ARVN units also worked the area. But these forces grew quickly after the arrival of the 1st Cavalry.

The company organization for air ambulances was unprecedented in Vietnam. The only other experience of an air ambulance company the 498th could draw on was that of the 421st Medical Company in Europe, which had its platoons, each consisting of six ships, scattered at four bases. Some pilots of the 498th wanted a similar dispersion while others preferred a centralized operation. Colonel Madrano told the Surgeon that he wanted to place a platoon each at Nha Trang, Qui Nhon, Pleiku, and Ban Me Thuot, the only secure bases in II Corps Zone that could possibly support them. All had inadequate resources to accept the entire company. Madrano soon dispersed his unit: 1 1/2 platoons at Qui Nhon; 1 1/2 platoons near the 52d Aviation Battalion at Pleiku; and the fourth platoon, along with the company headquarters, maintenance section, and operations section, at Nha Trang. Since the Qui Nhon contingent shared its compound with the 117th Aviation Company, some of the platoon's Medical Service Corps pilots had an opportunity to fly a few assault missions and learn about life as combat pilots. The technique the 117th taught was to fly out high, circle down steeply to the landing zone, and always keep the target in sight. This was a radical contrast to the techniques the 498th had practiced in Texas. The low-level approaches they had practiced at Camp Bullis had ill-prepared them for work in the mountainous Central Highlands of II Corps Zone.

When it first became operational on 20 September, the 498th was authorized only one-half the pilots it needed, so the USARV Surgeon and the 1st Logistical Command pitched in to help. Nonmedical commissioned and warrant officer pilots were sent on temporary duty to the 498th. Some of these men were at first reluctant to leave their gunships and transports, but toward the end of their term with the 498th most wanted to stay longer.

The distance of the deployed 498th platoons from their control headquarters in Saigon, the 1st Logistics Command, helped create a familiar problem. Each commander in II Corps Zone thought that some or all of the air ambulances belonged to him. Each thought that the authority to dispatch a flight should be his and that his isolated posts deserved individual Dust Off coverage. The problem was not alleviated by the assignment in late September of the 498th to the 43d Medical Group. Madrano had to exercise firmness to preserve the 498th's independence.

The disposition of his platoons compounded Madrano's problem of controlling his company. While the dispersion provided excellent air ambulance support to tactical combat units, it also created monumental problems for the company. Maintenance had to be carried on at three sites while the entire maintenance platoon was stationed at Nha Trang. Madrano was in the air constantly, visiting platoons or field sites, coordinating operations, and often flying hot missions from his three bases.

November turned out to be an especially trying month for

everyone in the 498th — pilots, crews, and maintenance men. On 11 November one of the aircraft flew from Qui Nhon to pick up a wounded South Korean soldier. At the landing zone, just as the medical corpsman finished loading the patient, enemy soldiers opened fire on the aircraft; one round hit the pilot in the neck. The copilot looked to his left, saw the pilot's bloody wound, and grabbed the controls. By now the North Vietnamese had begun to surround the aircraft. Drawing on all the power he could, with no regard for the torque meter, the copilot made a low-level takeoff straight at the enemy. The crew chief leaned out the open cargo door and used an M14 as a club. The aircraft returned to Qui Nhon and the pilot was rushed to an emergency room. He survived, and later returned to the United States to recover.

On the night of 11 November an aircraft of the 4th Platoon responded to an evacuation request from a South Korean unit west of Qui Nhon. Once over the landing zone they descended rapidly. Near the ground the windshield suddenly fogged over and neither pilot could see outside the cockpit. Before they could reorient themselves and halt their descent the helicopter crashed on a mountain and burst into flames. The copilot managed to pull the pilot from the wreck but the other crewmen perished. Both pilots suffered serious burns and were evacuated to Japan. The next morning a ground ambulance evacuated the Korean casualties.

The 436th Medical Company (Provisional)

The next air ambulance company set up in South Vietnam was drawn mainly from detachments already in the country. In April 1965 Lt. Col. James W. Blunt, the Surgeon of the U.S. Army Support Command, Vietnam, complained about the common practice of casualty evacuation by nonmedical aircraft. He planned an increase of at least two more air ambulance detachments in Vietnam to help counter this practice. The commander of the new 82d Medical Detachment suggested that he also create a control unit, possibly a provisional company, to command the proposed four air ambulance detachments. Later in the year Col. Ralph E. Conant, Colonel Blunt's successor, decided that such a control unit would indeed reduce the current confusion in III and IV Corp Zone medical evacuation caused by the wide dispersion of the four detachments and by their erratic communications. By November he had started planning for a provisional air ambulance company composed of four detachments, analogous to the four decentralized platoons of the 498th Medical Company.

On 1 December 1965 the Medical Company (Air Ambulance) (Provisional) was created from the old 57th and 82d Detachments, and the new 254th and 283d Detachments. The 43d Medical Group, which already commanded the 498th Medical Company, now took control of the provisional company. The company's mission was to supervise all aeromedical evacuation in III and IV Corps Zones. The unit's first commander, Maj. Glenn Williams, immediately asserted his authority by having the 57th Detachment removed from the operational control of the 145th Aviation Battalion and the 82d Detachment from the 13th Aviation Battalion. Believing his first complement of personnel inadequate to supervise four widely separated detachments, Williams pushed his superiors to expand his staff. On 1 April he received permission to form a company headquarters of two officers and six enlisted men, who would supervise 46 officers and 114 enlisted men. The company operated twenty-two helicopters (five each for the 57th and 82d Detachments, and six each for the 254th and 283d Detachments).

The creation of the provisional company was expected to improve the coordination of the air ambulance detachments. But company newsletters and personal letters from its men show that the new unit was not a success. Each detachment retained its own identity and tended to regard the company as just another headquarters in the chain of command. Major Williams also found, as had Colonel Madrano in the 498th, that the unique mission and problems of the air ambulance units required a battalion-size staff instead of a company headquarters. No doubt more lives could have been saved if an aggressive battalion safety officer had been available. More helicopters could have flown if a battalion maintenance officer had been able to coordinate and supervise the work of the young detachment maintenance officers. Although U.S. warehouses were full of the latest flight and safety equipment, the pilots and crew members were seldom able to obtain it, since a young officer with no supply training, representing a small detachment, had little chance of finding his way through the maze of supply channels.

But Major Williams was unable to set up more than a small provisional company headquarters. In September 1966 the Provisional Company was renamed the 436th Medical Detachment (Company Headquarters) (Air Ambulance) and attached to the 68th Medical Group, which had become operational in Vietnam on 1 March. This name lasted until May 1967 when the 436th was renamed the 658th Medical Company. With the arrival of the 45th Medical Company Air Ambulance) in July 1967, the 658th was deactivated and the 57th and 82d Detachments were attached to the 45th. The 283d moved to Pleiku and the 254th to Nha Trang. Overall, the experiment had failed.

ATTLEBORO

In late 1966 Operation ATTLEBORO, the largest combined

U.S.-South Vietnamese operation since the start of the war, gave the medical evacuation system its severest test so far in Vietnam. Over 20,000 allied soldiers were embroiled in a struggle with a large enemy force moving against objectives in Tay Ninh Province.

In October 1966 the *101st North Vietnamese Regiment* and two regiments of the *9th Viet Cong Division* began to move east from their sanctuaries along the Cambodian border. One of the regiments aimed at the Special Forces camp at Suoi Da, hoping to draw allied units into an ambush by the other *9th Division* regiments. By the end of November the 1st Infantry Division, the 173d Airborne Brigade, and elements of the 4th and 25th Infantry Divisions entered the struggle. Even while dealing the Communist forces a severe setback the allied forces suffered heavy casualties. Friendly losses were 155 killed and 494 wounded.

During ATTLEBORO the 436th Medical Company flew continuous missions. In two of the battles all the company's aircraft were in action. By the end of November the Dust Off helicopters had brought some 3,000 wounded, injured, and sick soldiers in from the field, aided for the first time by newly-installed hoists: winches that allowed soldiers to be lifted to hovering aircraft.[1] In the month-long operation the enemy hit fourteen Dust Off helicopters, heavily damaged seven, and destroyed one.

One serious problem in the coverage by the air ambulances marred an otherwise impressive performance. Each of the four U.S. combat units in ATTLEBORO controlled its own Dust Off aircraft. Since the medical regulating officers with each combat unit rarely coordinated their unit's Dust Off missions with the other dispatchers, the air ambulance with a unit in battle flew a great deal while the other aircraft flew very little or not at all. Corrections were clearly in order.

The Dust Off system soon, almost too soon, had a chance to show what it had learned in ATTLEBORO. On 8 January 1967 twenty U.S. and ARVN units launched Operation CEDAR FALLS by penetrating the Iron Triangle northwest of Saigon. Over the next nineteen days the allied combat units sealed off, searched out, and destroyed Communist camps and troop concentrations throughout the area, killing 720 enemy soldiers.

During the planning stages of the operation the commander of the 436th had talked with Army staff about the medical evacuation problems he had seen during ATTLEBORO. With the staff's help he was able to establish a control net for dispatching and following all the Dust Off aircraft in CEDAR FALLS. All Dust Off requests during the operation funneled through two central dispatch agencies. Two Dust Off detachments then divided the battlefield, each supporting the unit

---

[1] See Chapter IV for a description of the hoist and various litters.

within its area. Between flights, pilots regularly stayed some time at the regulating sites to help coordinate missions. Much wasteful duplication of effort was eliminated; the Dust Off system had been further improved.

The 45th Medical Company

During 1967 a new medical company, the 45th, brought in new equipment and pilots. In July 1966 the 44th Medical Brigade, which had become operational 1 May, asked the U.S. Army, Vietnam, to deploy another air ambulance company. Col. Ray L. Miller, brigade commander, noted that since January monthly medical evacuations in South Vietnam had risen from three thousand to over five thousand. Combat damage was taking a heavy toll on the Dust Off aircraft. But Miller's superiors decided to wait for the arrival of some new air ambulance units already scheduled for Vietnam. As an interim measure they assigned six nonmedical helicopters to the evacuation units, three for each of the two air ambulance companies. The 45th's deployment was postponed a year.

In March 1967 General Westmoreland told the Commander in Chief, U.S. Army, Pacific, that his theater needed 120 air ambulances but had only 64 on hand. Even if he received forty-nine more, to which the approved troop list entitled him, he would lack seven aircraft. In April the U.S. Army, Vietnam, informed U.S. Army, Pacific, that in light of its growing forces, it had taken several steps to reduce the shortage of air ambulances. Its stopgap measures included giving the 498th and 436th air ambulance companies more nonmedical aircraft, giving basic medical training to those assault and transport crewmen who might find themselves evacuating the wounded, and even designating certain aircraft in the airmobile assault units to carry a medical corpsman during attacks. Since he thought that these measures were makeshifts only, Westmoreland urged that the new air ambulance company and four detachments be shipped to South Vietnam as soon as possible.

By mid-1967 U.S. troop strength in South Vietnam approached 450,000, and General Westmoreland was asking for even more soldiers. U.S. Army, Vietnam, at last asked for another air ambulance company and four more helicopter ambulance detachments. If granted, this request would place a total of 109 air ambulance helicopters in South Vietnam.

In late May 1967 the 45th Medical Company (Air Ambulance), stationed at Fort Bragg, North Carolina, received notice that it would soon leave for Vietnam. It had been on deferred status since 1965 with twenty-five obsolete H–19 helicopters. Since the company was unable to acquire its last twelve authorized pilots before departure, it deployed without the pilots for one entire flight platoon; too many aviation units were forming and deploying for all to have their full complement of pilots. Before departing, the unit picked up twenty-five new UH–1H's with powerful Lycoming L–13 engines. These aircraft could be fitted with hoists for in-flight loading of the wounded, and they also carried new DECCA navigational kits. By 13 September the 45th was fully operational at Long Binh, about twenty kilometers northeast of Saigon. The airfield section leader kept some of his men busy building a heliport tower, and proved adept at scrounging. His crash rescue team soon had a bright red fire truck. He liberated a 3,000-gallon fuel bladder for JP–4 helicopter fuel and another with pumps for the aircraft washrack.

The 45th soon committed itself to giving twenty-four hour standbys at several bases around Saigon. One aircraft also gave daylight support to the Australians in the Saigon area. At Long Binh the company kept three standby aircraft for nearby evacuations and another for VIP or medical administration missions. From June through September alone, nine of the aircraft were damaged in combat. In October the 93d Evacuation Hospital started using the 45th to transfer most of its patients to a casualty staging facility near Tan Son Nhut, saving the injured the discomfort of riding in ground ambulances over the congested and dusty streets of Saigon.

The Buildup of 1967

Overall, this was a year of massive buildup for U.S. Army forces in Vietnam. Parts of I Corps Zone, until then a U.S. Marine Corps responsibility, went Army. U.S. Army, Vietnam, received not only the 45th Medical Company, but also four new air ambulance detachments. The Dust Off units already in Vietnam were moved to obtain better coverage for the newly deployed troops. The 54th Medical Detachment (Helicopter Ambulance) arrived at Chu Lai in the southern I Corps Zone in August, immediately began combat training with the 498th Medical Company, and became operational on 25 September 1967. It supported the Americal Division, the Army's largest. The southern I Corps Zone proved to be one of the most hotly contested in South Vietnam, and the 54th soon amassed an enviable record of honorable and dedicated support.

Other medical units followed. In October the 159th Medical Detachment (Helicopter Ambulance) arrived in Cu Chi, twenty kilometers northwest of Saigon with a mission to support all units in the area, but primarily the U.S. 25th Infantry Division. In November the 571st Medical Detachment (Helicopter Ambulance) joined the 254th at Nha Trang. It did not become operational until 2 January 1968, because the congestion in the ports delayed the unloading of its equipment. In December the 50th Medical Detachment (Helicopter Ambulance) arrived at its base at Phu Hiep, in the southwestern I

Corps Zone, and assumed responsibility for the 173d Airborne Brigade, the 28th ROK Regiment, and all other forces in the vicinity. The day after its helicopters arrived, the 50th went into action. By the end of December it had evacuated 644 patients, including 100 Koreans.

One of the more dramatic missions flown in this buildup phase of the war occurred on 18 October 1966 when a Dust Off craft from the 82d Detachment flew a hot mission near Vi Thanh in the Delta. As the crew approached the landing zone and slowed their ship, the enemy opened up with heavy and light automatic weapons fire from three sides. The ship broke off its approach and went around for another try. On the second attempt it took several more hits, some in the fuel cells. Its fuel quantity gauge registered zero and it departed for a safer landing site. After the first Dust Off had cleared the area, a transport helicopter tried to get in and pull out the casualties. As soon as it neared the ground the enemy took it under fire, killing the pilot outright. The aircraft crashed in some trees at the edge of the landing zone.

When they saw how hot the pickup site was, a second Dust Off crew decided to land some two hundred meters from the crashed transport. As they neared their new site they took one hit in the fuel cell. Another round hit the electronics compartment, popped half the overhead circuit breakers, destroyed the compass, and lit up the master warning lights. The crew landed anyway, but the patients would not come out to the ship since mortar rounds began hitting the area. So Dust Off flew out and struggled back to Vi Thanh for maintenance work.

A third Dust Off crew radioed a nearby gunship that they would like to follow him in after he prepared the landing zone to make the Viet Cong keep their heads down. The gunship started in with Dust Off following. Enemy fire wounded both crew members on the armed UH-1C, nicknamed the "Huey Hog," but Dust Off continued in and this time managed to land. As soon as they touched down the crew chief and medical corpsman jumped out and started loading casualties, even though the enemy harassed them with rifle and mortar fire. They loaded four litter and eleven ambulatory patients, and signaled the pilots to take off. The pilot drew on his maximum power as they flew out to safety.

Riverine Operations

Apart from the drama of even routine evacuations, the Dust Off pilots working the Delta in this phase of the war had to cope with a new problem—furnishing medical evacuation for the joint riverine operations conducted by the U.S. Navy's River Assault Flotilla One, Task Force 117, and the 2d Brigade of the Army's 9th Infantry Division. Medical support for waterborne forces usually went with them down the rivers. One company of the 9th Medical Battalion staffed an armored riverine landing craft that was specially fitted with five bunks for patients. A helipad on the troop carrier consisted of little more than steel runway matting welded over a framework of pipe. Starting in May 1967 similar armored troop carriers, besides their six Navy crewmen, housed a medical team consisting of a battalion surgeon, medical assistants, and a radio-telephone operator. The normal route of evacuation was from the battlefield to the troop carrier by helicopter, then further evacuation by helicopter to a surgical or evacuation hospital. So the armored troop carrier with its medical complement was similar to a battalion aid station, except that space on board the ship was extremely limited. The craft usually could not hold a patient more than thirty minutes, and only one of these medical troop carriers supported each battalion committed to action.

On 3 April 1967 representatives of the 44th Medical Brigade, the 9th Infantry Division Medical Battalion, the U.S. Navy Task Force 117, and the 436th Medical Detachment (Company Headquarters) met aboard the U.S.S. *Montrose,* the flagship of the Mobile Riverine Force, to discuss medical care and evacuation. The participants started to work out standard operating procedures for riverine aeromedical evacuations. One of the biggest early problems was evacuation of soldiers who were wounded on boats. Col. Robert M. Hall, MACV Surgeon, advocated a floating litter that one or two soldiers could propel through the water to move a casualty to a helicopter landing area on the riverbanks. Hoists could also be used to lift the patients directly from the assault boats. The Dust Off pilots of the 436th tried both these techniques.

In the summer of 1967 the 45th Medical Company took over from the 436th the direct support of the 9th Division. It also supplied field-standby aircraft for the division base at Dong Tam. To control these aircraft effectively, the division designated a Dust Off control officer who monitored radio traffic and regulated the dispatches. The 45th continued this mission until 22 December 1968, when the 247th Medical Detachment (Helicopter Ambulance) arrived to provide evacuation coverage for the Delta.

By early 1968 Dust Off pilots supporting riverine operations no longer had to land on a postage stamp in the middle of the river. Because of the long evacuation route and scarcity of hospitals deep in the Delta, the 9th Division received permission to make a hospital ship out of a self-propelled barracks ship, the U.S.S. *Colleton.* In December 1967 the *Colleton* sailed to Subic Bay Naval Base in the Philippine Islands, where her sick bay was enlarged. One month later she rejoined the forces in South Vietnam. Topside the ship had a helipad with enough space for one helicopter to land with another parked to the side. Navy radio-telephone operators controlled all ap proaches to this pad. Down a wide ramp was the triage area with six litter stations. On a lower level was the air-conditioned, two table surgical suite. The *Colleton* proved so successful as a hospital ship that the division got permission to convert a second vessel. In August 1968 the U.S.S. *Nueces* was outfitted as a 37-bed hospital ship, leaving the *Colleton* with the surgical mission.

Dak To

Toward the end of 1967, U.S. forces in II Corps Zone fought a series of battles that in retrospect seem to be little more than a prelude to the great Communist offensive in the spring of 1968. But one of them, the battle around Dak To in the Central Highlands, presented the Dust Off pilots and unit commanders with several new problems: coordinating medical evacuations for a rapidly expanding number of allied combat units, arranging for backhauls for the heavy casualties that often swamped the nearby 71st Evacuation Hospital at Pleiku, and coping with field pickups in rugged terrain concealed by high, triple-canopy jungle.

In August and September 1967 enemy operations in Pleiku Province had dwindled. The 4th U.S. Infantry Division in the area had experienced only scattered contacts with the enemy since July, an abnormally long lull in the fighting. But in October intelligence had detected large and unusual troop movements near the triborder region, west of the Special Forces camp at Dak To in Kontum Province, to the north of Pleiku Province. The terrain in this southwest portion of Kontum Province is steep, rocky, and covered with heavy bamboo and jungle. Only one second class road, Route 512, extended into this area, and at Fire Support Base Dak To II it became a single-lane, loose-surface trail. Dak To, a small town thirty-seven kilometers up National Highway 14 from Kontum, housed South Vietnamese CIDG forces and their U.S. advisers. Late in October the Special Forces troops were constructing a new base nineteen kilometers west of Dak To along Route 512; a battalion of the 4th Infantry Division furnished screening security. When alerted of the enemy movement, the 4th Division commander, Maj. Gen. William R. Peers, quickly arranged to have his screening battalion reinforced by the 173d Airborne Brigade. He also sent a 4th Infantry brigade headquarters and a second battalion to the area.

In early November North Vietnamese soldiers launched mass attacks on these forces, who retaliating strongly, were further reinforced by the 1st Brigade, 1st Cavalry Division. While trying to disengage and withdraw, the enemy committed the *174th North Vietnamese Regiment,* a reserve unit, to cover their retreat. This resulted in a bloody fight for Hill 875, which the American forces assaulted for four days before taking it. By the end of the fighting in the Dak To area on 1 December, the U.S. forces there were supporting six ARVN battalions.

At the start of the fighting on 1 November, a single Dust Off ship from the 283d Medical Detachment evacuated the first casualties from the clearing station of the 4th Medical Battalion at Dak To II back to the 71st Evacuation Hospital at Pleiku. The radio-telephone operator at the clearing station took evacuation requests over the 1st Brigade's tactical net and relayed them to the Dust Off ship. When the first casualties from a large fight with the enemy took place on 3 and early 4 November, the 283d ship had to call on help from transport helicopters, both for field pickups and the trip to Pleiku. The 283d also quickly field-sited several Hueys at Dak To from its new home at Pleiku Air Force Base. Even the gunships of the 52d Combat Aviation Battalion started flying noncritical patients from Dak To back to Pleiku at the end of the duty day. When the 173d Airborne entered the fighting on 8 November two platoons of the 498th Medical Company (Helicopter Ambulance), twelve helicopters in all, field-sited at Dak To to cover the 173d's casualties.

The surgeons in the six operating rooms of the 71st Evacuation Hospital often could not handle the large number of casualties. Surgical lag time grew dangerously long. On 11, 12, and 21 November an overflow of casualties forced the evacuation of the less seriously wounded to the 67th and 85th Evacuation Hospitals at Qui Nhon. The Air Force offered invaluable backhaul service at these times. After 21 November the Air Force placed its own casualty staging facility at Dak To for evacuation of serious and critical patients to Pleiku.

The mountainous terrain around Dak To and the 200-foot high, triple-canopy jungle made it necessary to use extraordinary methods on many of the field pickups. During the first eight days of November the 283d Detachment flew fifty-nine hoist missions. But the hoists only partly solved the problem; many patients in early November had wounds at least a day old before a doctor saw them. Nurses, corpsmen, and physicians had to quickly relearn the techniques of debriding wounds grown septic through delayed treatment. After the first week in November the ground units began using chain saws and plastic explosives to clear landing zones. Even though the plastic explosives and chain saws reduced the number of hoist missions, just one usually put the pilot and his crew in grave danger. During a night hoist on 13 November southwest of Dak To, one Dust Off aircraft took eighteen hits while at a stationary hover. A night hoist mission was undoubtedly the most unnerving kind of evacuation flight. Even if enemy resistance was slight, the technical problems of such a mission could take a heavy toll on a pilot's physical and mental well-being.

The battle for Hill 875 accounted for many of the casualties evacuated by Dust Off. For sixty hours only a few aircraft could reach the ground forces. In the middle of that period, Lt. Col. Byron P. Howlett, Jr., had four Air Force fighters and four helicopter gunships cover his approach to a small landing zone on the hill. He landed safely and loaded casualties, but on the way out with five seriously injured soldiers his ship took a hit in the rotor head. The ship struggled back to the 173d's clearing station and could not be flown out. After Colonel Howlett left the area, Maj. William R. Hill tried to get into the same landing zone but took fourteen hits and had to abort the mission. The next day the 173d secured the area around the landing zone and Dust Off evacuated 160 casualties. All in all, the Dust Off units had four aircraft shot up and five crewmen wounded while evacuating 1,100 patients. The system had proven resourceful enough to solve several new and perplexing problems.

The 54th and the Kelly Tradition

Pilots in any war consider themselves an elite group, and this was no less true for the Dust Off pilots in Vietnam than for the combat pilots. The Lafayette Escadrille of American pilots in France in World War I had set the pattern — a high life style and the *esprit de corps* possible in a small unit of highly skilled fighting men, in control of the most advanced technology. The dramatic entries of Dust Off ships into combat zones, usually unarmed and often unescorted, gave the pilots and crews a publicity that only heightened their sense of camaraderie. In the Korean War well-defined battle lines had permitted most helicopter medical evacuations to originate behind friendly lines. But the frontless nature of the guerrilla war in Vietnam demanded a novel marriage of the dash of the combat pilot with the often unheralded courage of the Army medical corpsman.

Maj. Charles L. Kelly was the first Dust Off pilot to exploit fully the possibilities of the medical helicopters. Not all Medevac and Dust Off pilots who arrived after his death tried to emulate his daring, but all fully understood that they could fly few of their missions without a good dose of raw courage. No Dust Off unit came closer to combining the Kelly tradition and the legacy of the Lafayette Escadrille than the 54th Medical Detachment (Helicopter Ambulance) stationed at Chu Lai, a port city on the southern coast of I Corps Zone.

In June 1967 the 54th was stationed at Fort Benning, Georgia, providing evacuation coverage for its Infantry, Airborne, and Ranger Schools. That month when the unit received an alert notice for deployment to Southeast Asia, only three of its members were eligible to go: Capt. Patrick H. Brady and two enlisted men. As new personnel began to filter into the unit, it also received six new UH–1H's straight from the Bell plant.

Captain Brady, who had flown with Kelly in 1964 and assumed

command of Detachment A at Soc Trang after his death, began training the new pilots. All the new warrant officer pilots came from the same flight school class that had graduated 6 June. All but one of their names began with "S." The Army had taken an entire alphabetical block out of the class and assigned it to the 54th. After introducing the pilots to the aircraft, Brady stressed his technique of tactical flying, which involved close analysis of the terrain to find the best approach to a hot landing zone.

The advance party, led by Brady, flew over to Vietnam early in August and reported to the 44th Medical Brigade at Long Binh. He was instructed to take his unit to Chu Lai in I Corps Zone. Flying north along the coast, they stopped off for a night to visit friends at the 498th Medical Company at Qui Nhon. Maj. Paul A. Bloomquist, commander, was not able to add much to the scanty information the 54th already had about its new assignment. At Chu Lai, Brady went to the 2d Surgical Hospital, which offered him a plot of land near the airfield. Most of the personnel and equipment of the 54th flew over on a USAF C-141 and arrived on 23 August. The 44th Medical Brigade assigned the 54th to the 55th Medical Group, which, in turn, gave operational control of the 54th to the 498th Medical Company.

As soon as all the men arrived, everyone pitched in to build a living area. Thanks to their industry and Brady's determination, they soon had a home. They obtained the first flush toilets in the Chu Lai area, even before the commanding general. Each man had a private room. They also built hot-water showers, a necessity in an area covered with red clay and dust. The enlisted men had a two-story rock-faced billet, which also contained the unit's music room, steam room, bar, and air-conditioned library, stocked by Captain Brady with 5,000 volumes. Outside was a pond, lined with palm trees and spanned by a wooden bridge. The unit's pets included several ducks, Gertrude the goose, Super Oink the pig, and Frances the monkey. Most of the men found themselves bicycles, and when Frances fell off one of them and hurt herself, the nearby 2d Surgical Hospital gladly restored her to health. For rest and relaxation, most of the men liked to go out to an island named Cu Lao Re, an extinct volcano that Navy men also used for scuba diving, fishing, and sunning.

When the U.S.N.S. *Card,* carrying the unit's helicopters and spare parts, arrived at Vung Tau, a port at the mouth of the Saigon River, on 24 September, the 54th's commander, Maj. Robert D. McWilliam, sent crews down to accept them, inspect them, and ferry them back to Chu Lai. The next day the unit became totally operational. To stagger personnel departure dates and provide some personnel continuity, it was customary to infuse a new unit in Vietnam with men who had already been in the country a few months, shifting some of the new men to older units. But the 54th resisted attempts to break up its original team. McWilliam and Brady knew the value of unit cohesion. They also instilled in their pilots the attitude that every mission, day or night, was urgent and should be treated as such, whether the patient was a papa-san with worms or an American soldier bleeding to death.

One day of the unit's work impressed all the people in the Chu Lai area. Friday, 29 September, became embedded in the memories of the 54th as "Black Friday." The day started out as usual — the crews eating breakfast, preflighting their ships, and then flying a couple of routine missions. But by that evening all six of the unit's aircraft had been subjected to intense enemy fire at various landing zones, and all had been damaged. Three crewmen had been wounded. This was a true baptism of fire for the fledgling unit. That night most of them looked out at the twelve months that stretched before them, and thought that it would be a very long year. In fact, twenty-two of the crewmen would be wounded during that year, but none killed.

Dust Off Wins Its First Medal of Honor

As Dust Off flew more and more missions the bravery of its pilots and crews became evident to all who fought in South Vietnam. While each of these pilots returned from a Dust Off mission something of a hero, some pilots distinguished themselves more than others. On the night of 5 January 1968 a South Vietnamese reconnaissance patrol left its camp in a heavily forested valley surrounded by mountains west of Chu Lai. An enemy force soon hit the patrol and inflicted several casualties. When the patrol limped back into camp with its wounded, Sgt. Robert E. Cashon, the senior Special Forces medical specialist at the base, tended to two critical patients and radioed his headquarters for a Dust Off ship. Soon the aircraft arrived overhead and tried several times to land in the camp. The pilot finally had to leave because fog and darkness obscured the ground. The monsoon season had enshrouded the mountains in soft, marshmallow clouds and fog several hundred feet thick. The clouds and fog extended east all the way to the flatlands between the mountain chain and the South China Sea.

Dawn brought little improvement in the weather. Visibility and ceiling were still zero. The next crew who tried to reach the camp, at 0700, also failed, even though they had been flying in that area for five months. True to the Kelly legacy of unhesitating service, Patrick H. Brady, now a major, and his crew of Dust Off 55 now volunteered for the mission into the fog-wrapped mountains.

They flew from Chu Lai to the mountains at low level just under the cloud base, then turned northward to Phu Tho where a trail wound westward through the mountains to the reconnaissance camp.

The fog grew so thick that none of the crew would even see the rotor tips of the helicopter. To improve the visibility, Brady lowered his side window and tilted his ship sideways at a sharp angle from the ground. The rotor blades blew enough fog away for him to barely make out the trail below the ship. Hovering slowly along the trail and occasionally drawing startled enemy fire, Dust Off 55 finally reached the valley and the camp. The visibility there was so poor that the ship completely missed the camp's landing zone and set down in a smaller clearing less than twenty meters square between the inner and outer defensive wires of the camp. The outpost had earlier taken mortar rounds and was still under sniper fire. Sergeant Cashon later said that the landing area would have been hazardous even in good weather. But Dust Off 55 loaded up, climbed out through the soup, and flew the two critical patients and four others to surgical care.

Brady's sweat from the first mission was hardly dry when another request chattered in over the 54th's radio. In the late afternoon of the day before, a company of the 198th Light Infantry Brigade, 23d Infantry Division, operating on the floor of the Hiep Duc Valley, came under a concerted attack by six companies of the *2d North Vietnamese Division.* For nine hours from their well-fortified positions in the surrounding hills, the North Vietnamese rained mortars and rockets on the Americans. The enemy had covered the likely flight paths into the area with 12.7-mm. antiaircraft guns. Early in the assault they had shot down two American gunships. Difficult communications and the nearness of the enemy on the night of the fifth had made a Dust Off mission impossible, even though the enemy had inflicted heavy casualties on the Americans. By dawn the company had sixty wounded on its hands.

On the morning of the sixth, a Dust Off pilot WO1 Charles D. Schenck, starting from fire support base West overlooking the valley, tried to fly a medical team out to the company and bring some of the wounded back. But the vertigo he suffered from the zero visibility forced him to abort. Shortly after he returned and told Dust Off Operations Control of his failure, Major Brady and Dust Off 55 began to prepare for flight. Brady, who knew the Hiep Duc Valley, listened to Schenck and the other pilots who had tried to reach the stranded company. Then he loaded a medical team in his ship, cranked the engine, and took off. Several miles from the battle area he found a hole in the soupy clouds through which he descended to treetop level. After twenty long minutes of low-level flight, Dust Off 55 neared the stricken company. Brady's surprise approach and the poor visibility threw off the enemy's aim; the helicopter landed safely.

Once on the ground the medical team quickly found and loaded the most seriously wounded. Brady made an instrument takeoff through the clouds, flew to fire base West, and delivered his casualties to the aid station. He then briefed three other crews on how he would execute his next trip into the area. The three ships tried to follow Brady in, but thick fog and enemy fire made them all climb out and return to West. Brady kept going, landed, picked up a load of wounded, and flew them out to West. Twice more he hovered down the trail and brought out wounded. Although the three other ships again tried to emulate his technique, none could make it all the way. Brady and his crew evacuated eighteen litter and twenty-one ambulatory patients on those four trips. Nine of the soldiers certainly would not have survived the hours which passed before the fog lifted.

As soon as Dust Off 55 refueled, Brady was sent on an urgent mission to evacuate the U.S. soldiers from a unit surrounded by the enemy twenty-six kilometers southeast of Chu Lai. Machine guns swept the landing zone as the North Vietnamese tried to wipe out the remaining American troops. Brady tried another surprise tactic. He low-leveled to the area, dropped in, turned his tail boom toward the heaviest fire to protect his cockpit, and hovered backward toward the pinned soldiers. The ship took rounds going in and once it was on the ground the fire intensified. For fear of being wounded or killed themselves, the friendly forces would not rise up and help load the casualties. Seeing this, Brady took off and circled the area until the ground troops radioed him in a second time. As he repeated his backward hover, the enemy tried once more to destroy the aircraft. But this time the ground troops loaded their comrades, who were soon in the rooms of the 27th Surgical Hospital at Chu Lai.

After four hours of flying that Saturday morning, Brady had to change his aircraft and find a relief copilot. A few hours earlier a platoon of the 198th Light Infantry Brigade on a patrol southeast of Chu Lai had walked into a carefully planned ambush. Automatic weapons and pressure-detonated mines devastated the platoon, killing six soldiers outright and wounding all the others. The platoon leader called for Dust Off. A helicopter soon landed, but took off quickly when a mine detonated close by, killing two more soldiers of the 198th who were crossing the minefield to aid the wounded.

Hearing this, Brady radioed that he would try the mission. The commander of the first aircraft suggested that Brady wait until the enemy broke contact. But Brady immediately flew out and landed on the minefield. Most of the casualties lay scattered around the area where they had fallen. Brady's crew chief and medical corpsman hustled the wounded onto the ship, disregarding the enemy fire and mines. As they neared the ship with one soldier, a mine detonated only five meters away, hurling the men into the air and perforating the aircraft with shrapnel holes. Both crewmen stood up, shaken by the concussion but otherwise unhurt, and placed the casualty on board. With a full load Brady flew out to the nearest hospital.

When he returned to the Dust Off pad at Chu Lai and delivered his patients, he again traded his ship for another. He flew two more urgent missions before he ended his day of glory well after dark. He had flown three aircraft and evacuated fifty-one wounded soldiers. For this day's work he was awarded the Medal of Honor.

Dust Off in the Saddle

As this buildup phase of the war ended in early 1968, U.S. troop strength in South Vietnam approached a half million uniformed men and women. By late 1967 the medical support required for this large military force and the supplementary medical support furnished to the South Vietnamese were fairly well-organized. Hospitals were rationally dispersed, and they usually performed their mission competently. Most of the air evacuation units that would serve in Vietnam were already there. Air crew casualties, while certainly disturbing, were not alarmingly high. The air ambulance helicopter had never been better equipped for its work. The advent of the Lycoming L-13 helicopter engine in the UH-1H's had eliminated the problem of the underpowered aircraft that would not always perform. The enemy's antiaircraft threat was still primitive, consisting mainly of eye-sighted small arms. The Army's new radios had smoothed communication difficulties considerably. And the hoist, while creating new dangers, enabled the Dust Off pilots and crews to extract casualties who otherwise would have languished hours before reaching a hospital.

Most important of all, the Kelly tradition had survived in full force in the 54th Detachment, and the pilots of the other detachments, the companies, and the divisional platoons often dared to enter landing zones that they suspected were dangerous. The courage of these pilots, far more than prescribed procedures and rigidly defined channels, had made the Dust Off system an object of reverence in the ever-shifting battlefields of Vietnam.

CHAPTER IV
The Pilot At Work

From 1965 to 1970 the U.S. Army in Vietnam perfected techniques of aeromedical evacuation that helped save the lives of hundreds of thousands of Americans and Vietnamese, both friend and foe, both soldiers and civilians. Many of the techniques had been worked out in the early years of U.S. involvement in Vietnam, from 1962 to 1965, when only the 57th and 82d Medical Detachments offered air ambulance service to the U.S. and South Vietnamese Armies. After the buildup of American forces began in 1965, the helicopters, procedures, and rescue equipment were improved and sometimes tested on mass casualties. Refinements of the system were made after the Tet offensive in 1968, and Army air ambulances evacuated more patients in 1969 than in any other year of the war. Then, as it began to withdraw its forces from Vietnam, the U.S. Army set up a training program to pass on its skills in air ambulance work to the South Vietnamese Army and Air Force. Assisting the development of the helicopters and rescue equipment and acquiring the skills needed to use them demanded exceptional imagination, dedication, and compassion, both of U.S. Army medical personnel and the South Vietnamese who learned from them.

The UH–1 Iroquois ("Huey")

When it entered the Vietnam War the U.S. Army lacked a satisfactory aircraft for medical evacuation. As early as 1953 the Aviation Section of the Surgeon General's Office had specified the desirable characteristics of an Army air ambulance. It was to be highly maneuverable for use in combat zones, of low profile, and capable of landing in a small area. It was to carry a crew of four and at least four litter patients, yet be easily loaded with litters by just two people. It had to be able to hover with a full patient load even in high altitude areas, and to cruise at least ninety knots per hour fully loaded. But in 1962 the Army's basic utility aircraft, the UH–1B made by Bell Aircraft Corporation, still did not meet these standards. It was, however, a small craft with a low profile, and the Army's MSC pilots could console themselves with the fact that the Huey was a far better air ambulance than the one their predecessors had flown in the Korean War. It had nearly twice the speed and endurance of the H–13 Sioux, and it could carry patients inside the aircraft, allowing a medical corpsman to administer in-flight treatment.

In almost all other respects it was less than perfect. One of its major problems was the comparatively low power of the engine. The critical factor in planning all helicopter flights with heavy cargoes is what pilots know as "density altitude" — the effective height above sea level computed on the basis of the actual altitude and the air temperature. The warmer the air, the less its resistance to the rotor blades and the less lift they produce. Because of its lack of fixed wings, which permit a powerless glide, a helicopter whose engine quits or fails to produce adequate power at a high density altitude can easily crash. Given enough forward airspeed and height, most helicopters, including all the Huey models, can drop to the earth and still land if the power fails, using the limited lift produced by the freely-spinning rotor blades. But this maneuver, called an autorotation, is virtually impossible to execute in a low-level, hovering helicopter. A writer for the Marine Corps suggests that this explains "...why, in generality, airplane pilots are open, clear-eyed, buoyant extroverts and helicopter pilots are brooders, introspective anticipators of trouble."

Although the A- and B-model Huey engine often lacked enough power to work in the heat and high altitudes of South Vietnam, it was much stronger than earlier Army helicopter engines. A great advance in helicopter propulsion had come in the 1950s with the adaptation of the gas turbine engine to helicopter flight. The piston-drive engines used in Korea and on the Army's UH-34 utility helicopters in the 1950s and early 1960s had produced only one horsepower for each three pounds of engine weight. The gas turbine engines installed on the UH-1 Hueys, which the Army first accepted in 1961, had a much more favorable efficiency ratio. This permitted the construction of small, low-profile aircraft that was still large enough to carry a crew of four and three litter patients against the back wall of the cabin. But the high density altitudes encountered in II Corps Zone in Vietnam meant that the UH-1A and UH-1B with a full crew — pilot, aircraft commander, crew chief, and medical corpsman — often could carry no more than one or two patients at a time.

In the early 1960s, shortly after the first U.S. Army helicopters were sent to South Vietnam, the Army began to use an improved version of the UH-1B: the UH-1D, which had a longer body with a cabin that could hold six litter patients or nine ambulatory patients. The longer rotor blade on the UH-1D gave it more lifting power, but high density altitudes in the northern two corps zones, where U.S. troops did most of their fighting, still prevented Dust Off pilots from making full use of the aircraft's carrying capacity. Finally in 1967 the commander of the 4th Infantry Division registered a complaint about his aeromedical evacuation support.

The 498th Medical Company, which served this area, had performed 100 hoist missions from July 1966 to February 1967 but had aborted 12 of them, 3 because of mechanical failures of the hoist and 9 because of the inability of the helicopter to hover. In March 1967 at Nha Trang, the staff of I Field Force, Vietnam, held a conference of various personnel involved in aeromedical evacuation in northern Vietnam. The conference noted the low engine power of the UH-1D's working in the Central Highlands, especially of those with the 498th Medical Company and the Air Ambulance Platoon of the 1st Cavalry.

In July 1967 the arrival at Long Binh of the 45th Medical Company (Air Ambulance), equipped with new, powerful UH-1H's marked the end to the Huey's propulsion problem. Headquarters, I Field Force, Vietnam, soon conducted a test of the engine power of the UH-1D, the Kaman HH-43 "Husky," and the new UH-1H with an Avco Corporation T-53-L-13 engine. The study showed that the maximum load of an aircraft hovering more than about twenty feet above the ground (out of ground effect) on a normal 95° F. day in the western Highlands was 184 pounds for the UH-1D with an L-11 engine, 380 pounds for the Husky, and 1,063 pounds for the UH-1H with an L-13 engine. This meant that on such a day the UH-1D could not perform a hoist mission; the Husky could pull at most two patients; and the UH-1H could pull five hoist patients. The L-13, rated at 27 percent more horsepower than the L-11, consumed 9 percent less fuel. The other air ambulance units in Vietnam obviously had to start using the UH-1H.

On 21 January 1968 the last UH-1D air ambulance in the U.S. Army, Vietnam, left the 57th Medical Department and became a troop transport in the 173d Assault Helicopter Battalion at Lai Khe. Now the entire fleet of air ambulances had powerful UH-1H's, solving many of the problems caused by high density altitudes, hoist missions, and heavy loads. Also, unlike most of the UH-1D's, the UH-1H's were fully instrumented for flight at night and in poor weather. They proved to be rugged machines, needing comparatively little time for maintenance and repairs. Like the earlier models, the H-models came with skids rather than wheels, to permit landing on marshy or rough terrain. The UH-1H's only important departure from the 1953 specifications of the Aviation Section was its inability to sustain flight if part or all of one rotor blade were missing. It was a single-engine craft with only two main rotor blades; the loss of all or part of one main blade would create an untenable imbalance in the propulsion system. And the Army version of the UH-1H had a flammable magnesium-aluminum alloy hull. Still, in most ways the UH-1H proved to be an ideal vehicle for combat medical evacuation.

The Hoist

The terrain in Vietnam — a mixture of mountains, marshy plains, and jungles — dictated the use of the helicopter for almost all transport. The changes in the design of the UH-1 Iroquois and its equipment during the Vietnam conflict stemmed largely from the problems presented by that difficult terrain. Early in the war the 57th Detachment recognized the need for some means of getting troops up to a helicopter hovering above ground obstacles that prevented a landing. The 57th sorely needed such a device for use in heavily forested areas, where until then medical evacuations had required moving the wounded and sick to an open area or cutting a pickup zone out of the jungle. During three military operations against the Viet Cong in War Zone D from November 1962 to March 1963, the South Vietnamese Army and their American advisers became acutely aware of this problem. The thick jungles in the area made resupply and medical evacuation by helicopter extremely difficult. Some of the South Vietnamese units carried their wounded for as long as four days before finding a suitable landing area for the UH-1A's. The problem was most acute when soldiers were wounded in the first few days of an operation, before reaching their first objective. This forced the ground commander either to delay his mission while sidetracking to a pickup zone, to carry the wounded with the assault column, or to leave the casualties behind with a few healthy soldiers for protection.

In attacking this problem, the armed services and their civilian contractors devised two fanciful and ultimately unsuccessful devices. Each entailed loading the helicopter while it hovered above the obstacles that surrounded the wounded below. The XVIII Airborne Corps at Fort Bragg devised a collapsible box-like platform that the ground troops were to strap to the upper reaches of a large tree. After the helicopter had dropped the platform to the soldiers on the ground, they would climb the tree, attach the platform, bring up the wounded, and wait while the helicopter moved into a hover just above the platform and the crew extended a rigid ladder four feet below the aircraft skids. Supplies would then be moved down and wounded or sick soldiers up the ladder. Tests revealed the absurdity of the device: wounded troops could hardly be moved to the top of a tree with ease, and the platform itself proved difficult to secure in the upper reaches of dense, multi-layered jungle.

A variation on this theme, the "Jungle Canopy Platform System," consisted of two stainless steel nets and a large platform. From the hovering helicopter the crew would unroll the nets onto the top of the jungle canopy, so that they intersected at midpoint; then the crew would lower the platform onto the intersection of the nets and signal the pilots to land on it. Troops and supplies could then move to and from the aircraft. The 1st Cavalry Division tested the device in Vietnam during noncombat operations; actual combat reports on it could not be obtained because no unit would use it under those conditions. Without the platform the nets worked well for deploying troops but proved unreliable for other uses, such as medical evacuation. The test report concluded: "Based on commanders' reluctance to use the system, there appears to be no current requirement for the Jungle Canopy Platform System."

Despite these two failures, the Army did develop a piece of supplemental equipment for the Huey that both advanced the art of medical evacuation and placed extraordinary new demands on the air ambulance pilots: the personnel rescue hoist. The hoist was a winch mounted on a support that was anchored to the floor and roof of the helicopter cabin, usually just inside the right side door behind the pilot's seat. When the door was open, the hoist could be rotated on its support to position its cable and pulleys outside the aircraft, clear of the skids, so that the cable could be lowered to and raised from the ground. After a UH–1 was outfitted with the necessary electrical system, the aircraft crew could quickly install or remove the hoist. On a hoist mission, while the aircraft hovered, the medical corpsman or crew chief would use the hoist cable to lower any one of several types of litters or harnesses to casualties below. If a wounded soldier and his comrades were unfamiliar with the harness or litter, the crew chief would sometimes lower a medical corpsman with the device; then the hoist would raise both the medic and the casualty to the helicopter. The standard hoist eventually installed on the UH–1D/H could lift up to 600 pounds on one load and could lower a harness or litter about 250 feet below the aircraft.

As early as November 1962 the Surgeon General's Office had said that the Army's air ambulances needed a hoisting device. Under further pressure from the 57th Medical Detachment, the Surgeon General had the Army contract with Bell Aircraft Corporation and the Breeze Corporation for the personnel rescue hoist. The U.S. Army Medical Test and Evaluation Activity experimented with the new hoist at Fort Sam Houston in April and May 1965 and recommended that it be adopted with minor modifications.

In May 1966 the first hoists began arriving in Vietnam, and on 17 May, Capt. Donald Retzlaff of the 1st Platoon, 498th Medical Company, at Nha Trang, flew the first hoist mission in Vietnam. But within a week the hoist proved unreliable, prone to jam and break during a lift. After being grounded for two months for repairs and redesigning, the hoist, now modified, went back into service. It continued to be a maintenance problem for the rest of the war, but it functioned well enough to save several thousand lives.

Although air ambulance pilots began to use the hoist in Vietnam in August 1966, their commanders soon complained about the extraordinary hazards it brought to their work. The UH–1D was already burdened with a heavy single sideband (high frequency) radio and a navigation system; the extra weight of the hoist compounded the problem of the underpowered L–11 engine. Since the crew chief worked on the same side of the aircraft as the hoist, the helicopter was heavily overweighted on one side, and a strong gust of wind from the other side could endanger the craft's stability. The operation also demanded great strength and concentration of the pilots, especially if winds were gusting or if trees or the enemy forced a downwind or crosswind hover. The danger of mechanical troubles was obvious: almost by definition no emergency landing site was nearby, and even if it were, the ship usually was hovering at a height that precluded an autorotational touchdown in an emergency.

Adding to the tenseness of such a mission, the crews knew that the most vulnerable target in the war was a helicopter at a high hover. The precautions that had to be taken against sudden enemy fire proved especially taxing on the pilots. The men in the rear of the aircraft cabin would set the intercom switches on their helmets to "hot mike," allowing them to communicate with the rest of the crew without depressing their microphone buttons. While working the hoist or putting down suppressive fire the crew chief and medical corpman could keep the pilot informed of his nearness to trees or other hazards. While listening to this chatter, the pilots also had to be in radio contact with the people on the ground. In December 1966 an officer of the 1st Cavalry Division in the Central Highlands complained:

We are very dissatisfied with the hoist and any of its associated equipment. Mainly because we've been shot up pretty badly twice during Operation THAYER while in position for hoist extraction. Fortunately so far we've had only two crew members slightly wounded. On both occasions the VC haven't fired a shot in the last ten to thirty minutes. Then, just as the hook enters the pickup site, he cuts loose. He is so close to our troops on the ground ... the armed escort ships can't fire for fear of hitting our own troops.

The hook on the end of the hoist cable could accept several types of rescue devices. A traditional rescue harness worked well for pulling up lightly injured soldiers, but it proved difficult and often impossible to lower through the thick upper vegetation of Vietnam's forests and jungles. Seriously wounded soldiers usually had to be placed in the rigid wire Stokes litters and raised horizontally; but this too caused problems in thick jungles and forests. For the lightly wounded and the less seriously wounded, the air ambulances almost always used a device designed early in the war — a collapsible seat called the forest penetrator, which could easily be lowered through dense jungle canopy. Developed by the Kaman Corporation, the penetrator weighed twenty pounds, and had three small, paddle-like seats that could be rotated upwards to lock into place against the sides of the penetrator's narrow, three-foot long, bullet-shaped body. Once to the ground, the seats could be lowered and the wounded strapped on with chest belts. Although the version accepted by the Army had no protection for the casualty's head as he was raised up through the foliage, this seldom proved a problem. The first eight forest penetrators arrived in Vietnam in mid-June 1966, but extensive testing of the device with the new hoists was delayed until September and October. Medical personnel then found the device satisfactory and it became the normal means of lifting a conscious casualty. Unconscious soldiers were often lifted head up, in a device known as the semi-rigid litter: a flexible canvas jacket with a lining of wood straps and a rigid head cover.

Even when the penetrator was used, a hoist mission took considerably longer than usual at the pickup zone. Pilots flying the first missions found their ships often subject to accurate enemy fire. On 1 November 1966 the 283d Detachment at Tan Son Nhut got a request from a ground unit not far outside Saigon's noise and bustle. The unit had casualties deep under the jungle and needed a hoist to get them out. In the 283d, Capt. James E. Lombard and 1st Lt. Melvin J. Ruiz had the only ship fitted with a hoist.

As soon as they left the ground at Tan Son Nhut they radioed the ground unit and asked whether it had any gunships standing by or had asked for any. The unit answered that it had requested them but had no idea how long they would take getting there. Three minutes later Lombard and Ruiz arrived over the pickup site. Lombard told the troops on the ground that he would have to have gunship support before he could land. He radioed a gunship unit at Bien Hoa, a five minute flight away, and asked them to launch a team to cover his mission. He was told there would be a thirty minute delay. The ground unit commander than started a sales pitch: there had been one sniper, but they had got him, the area was secure now, they had two critically wounded. Lombard agreed to come down.

The ground unit popped a smoke grenade, and the Dust Off ship came to a hover over the spot where wisps of colored smoke drifted up through the trees. The crew chief played out the hoist cable. The forest penetrator was ten feet below the skids when an automatic weapon opened up on the helicopter from the right side. Bullets whined and zinged through the aircraft, and the pilot's warning lights lit up like a Christmas tree. Lombard broke off the hover. The hydraulics were gone and the crew heard crunching and grumbling sounds from the transmission. They headed east toward a safe haven at Di An, a four minute flight away. Suddenly the engine quit. Luckily within reach of their glide path lay an open area to which they shot an autorotation. With the controls only half working, Lombard had to make a running landing, skidding along the ground. The ship tipped well forward on its skids then rocked back to a stop. The engine compartment was on fire. The crew got out as fast as possible, the pilots squeezing between the door frame and their seats' sliding armor side plates, which were locked in the forward position. They started to run from the aircraft when they realized that their rifles and ammunition were still inside. The medical corpsman dashed back inside, grabbed the rifles and bandoliers, jumped back out, and distributed the arms.

They looked around and decided that they had overflown the enemy, who now separated them from the friendly unit with the casualties. Rather than head into a possible ambush, they started toward a knoll in the direction of Long Binh. Unknown to them, another platoon of the friendly company was out on a sweep headed in their direction. On the ground the crew was completely out of their environment. Their loaded M16's cocked on automatic, they were ready to shoot the first blade of grass that moved. Suddenly they heard the thump, thump, thump of troops running toward them. They stopped, waited, then saw U.S. troops coming at them through the bush.

They all went back to the landing zone, where they set up a small defensive perimeter. Later that afternoon, the platoon that had called in the request cut its way out of the jungle and joined them. Its two wounded had died on the way out. The company commander radioed Di An and asked its mortars to start laying a protective barrage around the perimeter. The first salvo landed on the company and wounded many of them. The commander radioed for another Dust Off. Two hours later as dusk approached, a Dust Off ship from the 254th Detachment flew in with a gunship escort. In several trips it evacuated nineteen wounded soldiers, the two dead, and the crew from the 283d. Lombard and Ruiz had flown the first of many hoist missions that resulted in the downing of an air ambulance. But the hoist had clearly added a new dimension to utility of the helicopter in Vietnam. Despite the new danger it brought to their work, the air ambulance crews responded with courage and dedication.

Evacuation Missions

Air ambulances received their missions either aloft in the aircraft, at the ambulance base, or at a standby base, usually near or at a battalion or brigade headquarters. The coverage given by the ambulances was either area support (to all allied units in a defined area) or direct support (to a particular unit involved in an operation). Direct support, in effect, dedicated the aircraft to a particular combat unit, and it usually relieved the aircraft commander of the need to receive mission authorization from his operations officer. Both air ambulances organic to combat units and nonorganic aircraft flew direct support missions.

Most air ambulance missions, however, originated during area support. An American or allied patrol would take casualties, usually in daylight, from enemy sniper fire, mines, or other antipersonnel devices. The patrol commander and medical corpsman would decide whether the casualties needed to be evacuated by helicopter. If a Dust Off or Medevac aircraft were needed, the patrol would, if its radio were powerful enough, send its request directly to the air ambulances or their operations control. If this were not possible, the patrol would use its tactical radio frequency to send the request back to its battalion headquarters. Whichever method was used, the request had to contain much information: coordinates of the pickup site, the number and types (litter or ambulatory) of patients, the nature and seriousness of the wounds or illness, the tactical radio frequency and call sign of the unit with the patients, any need for special equipment (such as the hoist, whole blood, or oxygen), the nationality of the patients, visual features of the pickup zone (including any smoke, lights, or flares to be used by the ground unit), the tactical security of the pickup zone, and any weather or terrain hazards. The first four elements were critical: with them a mission could be flown; without them no air ambulance could guarantee a response.

Two elements of any request were open to considerable interpretation by the ground commander and his medical corpsmen: the seriousness of the medical problem and the security of the pickup zone. Three levels of patient classification were used: urgent, priority, and routine. Urgent patients were those in imminent danger of loss of life or limb; they demanded an immediate response from any available air ambulance. Priority patients were those with serious but not critical wounds or illness; they could expect up to a four-hour wait. In theory a medical corpsman had to ignore the suffering of a patient in determining his classification: a soldier in great pain, with a foot mangled by a mine, warranted, if his bleeding were stanched, only a priority rating. In practice, despite the considerable efforts of aeromedical personnel, any patient bleeding or in great pain usually received an urgent classification. Just as many patients were overclassified, many dangerous pickup zones were reported as secure, and this too was understandable. Although some air ambulance units tried to fight the policy, Army doctrine limited the ground unit's responsibility in reporting on a pickup zone: if the unit's soldiers could safely stand up to load the casualties, the pickup zone could be reported as secure. So the air ambulance crew could never be sure that the airspace more than ten feet above the ground would be safe. It was highly important for an aircraft commander approaching a pickup zone to establish radio contact with the ground unit and learn as much as possible about enemy forces near the zone.

If the ground unit with the patient had to send its evacuation request through its battalion headquarters, the headquarters would make sure the request had all essential information and then either send it directly over the established air ambulance radio frequency or, if it lacked the proper radios, forward it to brigade headquarters, who almost always could communicate directly with the air ambulance operations officer.

Once an air ambulance received an urgent request, its personnel dropped any priority or routine tasks and headed toward the pickup zone. The aircraft commander performed a variety of duties of such a mission. He supervised the work of the pilot and two crewmen, and worked as copilot and navigator. En route he monitored both the tactical and air ambulance frequencies, and talked to the ground unit with the patient. Once over the pickup zone, he surveyed the area and decided whether to make the pickup, with due regard to urgency, security, weather, and terrain. If he decided to land he had to choose directions and angles of approach and takeoff. If problems developed at the pickup zone he had to decide whether to abort the mission. Once the pickup was made, he had to choose and receive confirmation on the suitability of a destination with medical facilities. He usually sat in the left front seat, leaving the right seat to the pilot, who needed a view of the hoist on the side and the flight control advantages of the right side position. Usually the commander left the en route flying to the pilot, but sometimes flew the final approach and the takeoff, especially at an open pickup zone. During a hover on a hoist mission he and the pilot alternated on the controls every five minutes.

This practice of flying with two pilots originated in the early days of U.S. military involvement in Vietnam. Since the Korean War, helicopter detachments had flown with one pilot in the cockpit. The transportation aviation units which were in Vietnam when the 57th medical detachment deployed there in 1962 already had made it a policy to fly their H-21's with two pilots in the cockpit. There were convincing reasons. If a solo pilot were wounded or killed by enemy gunfire his crew and ship would probably be lost, but a second pilot could take over the controls. A solo pilot also stood a good chance of getting lost over the sparsely populated Vietnamese countryside, where seasonal changes in precipitation produced great changes in the features of the terrain, making dead reckoning and pilotage difficult even for a pilot with excellent maps and aerial photographs. A second pilot could act as a navigator en route to and from a pickup zone.

The 57th quickly learned the value of two-pilot missions and asked for authorization to fly them. The denial they received referred to the official operator's manual for the UH-1, which said that the helicopter, although equipped for two pilots, could be flown by one. Nevertheless, with seven aviators and only four aircraft, and one of those usually down for maintenance, the 57th usually flew their missions with two pilots up front. All the air ambulance units that followed adopted this practice, and eventually they obtained authorizations to do so.

Besides the two pilots, an air ambulance usually carried a crew chief and medical corpsman. The crew chief's most important preflight duty was preventive maintenance: keeping the aircraft flightworthy through proper and timely inspections and repairs. He also had to make sure that the aircraft had all essential tools, equipment, and supplies on board. The medical corpsman's only vital preflight duty was to supply the craft with the small amount of medical supplies that could be used in the short time taken by most evacuation flights: a basic first aid kit, morphine, intravenous fluids, basic resuscitative equipment, and scalpels and tubes for tracheostomies. At the pickup zone the crew chief and corpsman often worked together to load the casualties. If the hoist had to be used, one of them would operate it on the right side of the aircraft while the other stood in the opposite door, armed with a rifle to suppress enemy fire and to see that the aircraft stayed at a safe distance from obstacles. Once the patients were loaded, the crew chief helped the corpsman give them medical aid.

The standard operating procedure of an air ambulance unit usually required one aircraft crew to be on alert at all times in "first up" status, ready to respond immediately to an urgent request. Like all ambulance crews, the men sprang into action as soon as the siren in their lounge went off. Most units practiced often to cut the precious minutes needed to get their aircraft, warm the engine, and lift off. Many could get off in less than three minutes, unless the unit commander demanded a certain amount of preflight planning. Once aloft, the aircraft commander would open his radio to the Dust Off frequency and receive his assignment from the radio operator back at the base.

He then turned the ship toward his objective, and at some point en route switched to the tactical frequency of the ground unit with the casualties. This allowed him to reassure the unit that help was on the way, assist the medical aidman on the ground in preparing for the evacuation, and check with the ground commander on dangers from the terrain, weather, or enemy. The method of approach to the pickup zone varied. Some units specified a standard approach, such as a steep, rapid descent from high altitude. But some of the most respected commanders believed in letting the aircraft commander use the many variables of the situation to determine the fastest, safest means of getting down to the wounded.

On the ground the medical corpsman and the crew chief usually left the aircraft, put the patients on litters, and loaded them onto the ship. About half the time the casualty would not have received any medical treatment before he reached the air ambulance. When the hoist first went into operation, medical personnel publicized it and offered training in its use to ground combat and medical personnel. This reduced the likelihood that the medical corpsman would have to be lowered during a hoist mission to help load the patients, allowing either the corpsman or the crew chief to put down suppressive fire while the other lowered and raised the hoist cable. A few units, especially the organic air ambulances, routinely carried a fifth crewman during a hoist mission—a gunner to protect the ship, its crew, and its casualties.

Once the patients were aboard and safely secured, the pilot took off. The corpsman tried to find and treat the most serious patient, and report the nature of the problem to the aircraft commander. The decision on where to fly the patients then entered the medical regulating network. The aircraft commander radioed the nearest responsible medical regulating officer, who confirmed or altered the commander's choice of destination. This choice was based on the commander's knowledge of the specialized surgical capabilities of the hospitals in his area and on his daily morning briefing as to the current surgical backlog in these hospitals. Standard practice was to take the most serious patient directly to a nearby hospital known to have all the equipment and care he immediately needed. If that hospital then determined that he needed more sophisticated care than it could offer, he was backhauled as far to the rear as possible. A secondary objective was to take the patient to the hospital in the area that had the smallest surgical backlog, to reduce the time between wounding and the start of surgery. The supporting medical group in each area of operations usually assigned, at least after 1966, a forward medical regulating officer to each combat brigade headquarters, and those regulators kept aware of the most current surgical backlogs in all nearby hospitals. Since they had more current information on surgical backlogs than the aircraft commanders, the regulators had the authority to change the commander's choice of destination.

Since most pickups were made within range of a surgical, field, or evacuation hospital, the ambulances usually overflew the battalion aid stations and division clearing stations, which could offer only basic emergency treatment that was already available on the helicopter, and deposited the patients at a facility that offered definitive resuscitative treatment. Although the less serious patients often found themselves overevacuated, the practice saved thousands of patients who demanded immediate life-saving surgery.

The effective functioning of an air ambulance depended heavily on its bank of four radios: FM, UHF, VHF, and single sideband (high frequency). The FM radio contained the frequencies of the Dust Off operations center, the tactical combat unit, and most hospitals. VHF and UHF were infrequently used. And the single sideband contained the medical regulating frequencies. The ambulance would usually stay on its Dust Off frequency for flight following until he approached the pickup zone, when it would switch over to the tactical frequency of the unit with the casualties. After the pickup the ambulance would switch briefly to the frequency of the forward medical regulator, which was closely monitored by his group medical regulating officer. Then the ambulance would switch back to the Dust Off frequency for flight following until it approached the hospital, when it would switch to the hospital's frequency, usually on the FM radio, to warn the doctors of the approach.

Although most of these procedures for area support missions also applied for direct support missions, there were a few important differences. Early in the war the 57th and 82d Medical Detachments, under the operational control of aviation battalions in the Delta, flew many such missions. The battalions would warn the detachments of planned airmobile operations and their requirements for aeromedical support. During a combat insertion, one or more Dust Off ships orbited near the landing zones at two or three thousand feet, out of effective small arms range, with the pilots monitoring the helicopter-to-ground talk on the FM band, helicopter gunship talk on UHF, and any airplane-to-gunship talk on VHF. If a patient pickup became necessary during a ground fight, the command-and-control helicopter of the flight would designate two gunships to accompany the Dust Off ship into and out of the area. The gunships would switch over to the Dust Off frequency and make a slow pass over the area to draw fire, find the source, and suppress it. Then Dust Off would go in covered by the gunships. Later in the war organic air ambulances sometimes accompanied the flight of transport helicopters into the landing zones, and stood by waiting for casualties. More often they orbited the area of operations or stood by at the nearest battalion or divisional clearing station. While affording excellent aeromedical coverage for the supported unit, direct support missions limited the ability of the air ambulances to respond to emergencies elsewhere.

Evacuation Problems

All helicopter pilots in Vietnam had to cope with problems for which they might be unprepared or poorly equipped. By the nature of their work, air ambulance pilots experienced such problems more often than transport and gunship pilots. Except for the Medevac helicopters of the 1st Cavalry Division, the air ambulances carried no armament heavier than the pilots' M16 rifles, and most of the air ambulance missions were executed by a single ship rather than a well-prepared team, known as a "gaggle." Soldiers were shot and injured without regard to the terrain or weather, and the air ambulances were expected to make their way to the casualties as soon as possible. The poor navigation equipment on the Hueys and the shortage of instrument-trained pilots early in the war exacerbated the difficulty of coping with South Vietnam's weather. While maintenance problems plagued all the helicopter crews in South Vietnam, the special demands of air ambulance work, such as hoist missions, compounded the problems. Speed was important to inbound as well as outbound flights, making stops for refueling a dangerous luxury. While few of these problems could be totally solved, the air ambulance units often found ways to minimize them. When refueling during a mission could not be avoided, the unit often called ahead to an established fuel depot and made an appointment for refueling at an en route landing strip. When a unit was jointly based with a gunship battalion, arrangements could sometimes be made for an armed escort, especially on a hoist mission.

One of the problems that persisted throughout the war was the expectation that the air ambulances would transport the dead. Nothing in USARV regulations authorized the ambulances to carry the dead; but both ARVN and American soldiers expected this service. Nonmedical transport helicopters and gunships often evacuated both the dead and the wounded. If Dust Off ships had routinely refused to carry the dead even when they had extra cargo space, the combat units might have decided to rely exclusively on their transports and gunships to evacuate both the wounded and the dead, resulting in a marked decline in the care provided the wounded. Combat operations might also have suffered, for ARVN soldiers often would not advance until their dead had been evacuated. So most air ambulance units practiced carrying the dead if it did not jeopardize the life or limb of the wounded.

The language barrier also hampered the work of the air ambulance crews. Almost one-half the sick and wounded transported by the air ambulances could not speak English, and the crews usually could not speak enough Vietnamese, Korean, or Thai to communicate with their passengers. Early in the war USARV regulations prohibited a response to an evacuation request unless an English-speaking person were at the pickup site to help the air ambulance crew make its approach and evaluate the patient's needs, or unless the requesting unit supplied the air ambulance an interpreter. But the scarcity of good interpreters in the South Vietnamese Army meant that Dust Off evacuated many Vietnamese whose needs were only vaguely understood. Even when the air ambulance unit shared a base with an ARVN unit, the language problem proved serious. A former commander of the 254th Detachment remembered such an experience:

The periodic attacks on the airfield were experiences to behold. Trying to ge from our quarters to the airfield was the most dangerous. The Vietnamese soldiers responsible for airfield security didn't speak English and with all the activity in the night—vehicles driving wildly about, people on the move, machine gun fire and mortar flares creating weird lighting and shadows—the guards were confused as to who should be allowed to enter the field and who had no reason to enter. If one could get to the field before the road barriers and automatic weapons were in place all was well. Later than that, one might just as well not even try to get on the field. We had several instances of the guards turning our officers back at gunpoint! We tried to get ID cards made but the Vietnamese refused to issue any cards. We sometimes felt we were in more danger trying to get to the airfield during alerts than we were picking up casualties.

The pilots and crews also had to contend with the ever-present danger of a serious accident. Until later in the war most of the pilots lacked the instrument skills needed to cope with the poor visibility typical of night missions and weather missions. The DECCA navigation system installed in the UH-1B's and UH-1D's proved virtually useless early in the war. More pilots died from night- and weather-induced accidents than from enemy fire.

To cope with this danger, most of the pilots new to Vietnam quickly learned the virtue of a cool head and even a sense of humor. One former commander of a unit recalled the day that his alert crew at Qui Nhon received a request for the urgent evacuation of an American adviser who had fallen into a punji trap. (Such traps held sharpened wood stakes driven into the ground with the pointed ends facing up, often covered with feces, onto which the victims would step or fall.) It was late afternoon, approaching dusk, but Maj. William Ballinger and his pilot scrambled on the emergency call. They flew down the coast then turned inland to the pickup point. The casualty turned out to be a Vietnamese lieutenant with no more than a rash. Since they were already there, the crew picked him up and started back to Qui Nhon.

On the way down the weather had turned bad, and when they headed north rain began. Night fell and the rain grew worse. Wondering whether they should set down or continue, they called the Qui Nhon tower operator and asked for the local weather. The operator reported a 3,000 foot ceiling and five miles visibility. The pilots thought they were in the middle of an isolated storm and they expected to break out shortly. After flying on and still not clearing the storm, they radioed the tower again and got the same report. Now their visibility was so bad they had to drop low and fly slowly up the beach. As they passed a point they knew to be only five miles from Qui Nhon, with the rain still pelting down, they again radioed the tower operator and got the same report: ceiling, 3,000 feet and five miles visibility. Ballinger asked for the source of the weather report, and the operator replied, "This is the official Saigon forecast for Qui Nhon." Ballinger told the man to look outside the tower and then tell him what the weather was. The operator replied, "Oh, sir, you can't see a damned thing out there." The pilots had to fly low and slow to the base and were relieved when their skids touched the runway. Only then could they indulge in a good laugh.

Night missions quickly became a major problem in themselves. The difficulties of such missions in a rural society were obvious: roads and population centers rarely were well lighted enough to aid in navigation to a pickup zone; terrain, especially in mountainous areas, became a great danger to ambulances that lacked adequate navigation instruments; and adequate lighting at the pickup zone rarely existed. In the dry season a landing light reflecting off the dust thrown up by the rotorwash could quickly blind a pilot just before touchdown. Throughout the war a considerable number of pilots and commanders refused to fly night missions or else flew them only for urgent cases. Others, however, thought that night flying offered many advantages that at least compensated for its problems. A few, such as Patrick Brady, even preferred night missions.

Early in the war the 57th Detachment routinely flew night evacuations, so much so that at one staff meeting General Stilwell, the Support Group commander, asked why the 57th could fly so well at night when few others could or would. He quickly learned that one of the aids used by the 57th was the AN/APX–44 transponder, which allowed Air Force radar stations to follow the aircraft at night or in bad weather and vector them to and from a pickup site. Early in 1964 General Stilwell charged the medical detachment with the task of conducting a test on the feasibility of making combat assault insertions at night. In the Plain of Reeds the pilots experimented with parachute flares, tested the available radio and navigation equipment, and concluded that although night missions were suitable for medical evacuation they were not suitable for combat assaults.

Night missions called for a few specialized techniques. En route at night to a pickup zone an air ambulance would fly with either its external rotating beacon or position lights on. Once below 1,000 feet on its approach to the zone, it would douse these lights and dim its interior instrument panel lights as soon as the ship drew within range of enemy fire. About five hundred feet from the touchdown, the pilot would briefly turn on his landing light to get a quick look at the pickup zone. Then he would douse the landing light until the last 200 feet of the approach. In an article in *Army Aviation Digest,* Capt. Patrick Brady recommended a final descent at right angles to the ground unit's signal, since a pilot could see much better through the open side window than through the windshield, especially one covered with bulletproof plexiglass. On the ground the soldiers would use flashlights, small strobe lights, or vehicle headlights to mark the pickup zone. Some lights, such as flares, burning oil cans, and spotlights, tended to blind the pilot on final approach. A pilot in contact with soldiers on the ground would try to warn them of this early enough to allow a change of lights if necessary. On takeoff the lighting sequence on the ambulance would be reversed.

While night magnified the dangers of weather and terrain, Captain Brady correctly noted that it reduced the danger of enemy fire. Although the enemy would always hear the approach of the noisy Huey, he could rarely see it in the dark. An exhaust flame or the moonlight would sometimes betray a blacked-out aircraft, but the enemy could rarely direct accurate fire at the ship. Only night hoist missions allowed the enemy to get an accurate fix on an air ambulance, and the extreme hazards of hovering an aircraft close to ground obstacles at night made even the best air ambulance pilots avoid such missions unless a patient were in imminent danger of loss of life.

A scarcely less dangerous form of night mission, a night pickup in the mountains in bad weather, was also beyond the capacity of most air ambulance pilots. Brady, however, developed a technique for such a mission that made it feasible if not safe for a highly competent pilot. One night in the fall of 1967, in Brady's second tour in Vietnam, his unit, the 54th Detachment at Chu Lai, received a Dust Off request from a 101st Airborne Division patrol with many casualties in the mountains to the west. Heavy rains and fog covered the area, and after a few attempts Brady decided that he would never get to the casualties by trying to fly out beneath the weather. He would have to come down through the fog and rain with the mountains surrounding him. He took his aircraft up to 4,500 feet and vectored out to the mountains on instruments. As he approached the mountains he took his ship up to 7,000 feet. From his FM homing device he knew when he was directly over the pickup site. Then he radioed an Air Force flare ship in the area and asked its pilot to meet him high above the pickup zone and foul weather below. The Air Force pilot agreed and at Brady's suggestion took his plane to 9,000 feet directly overhead and began to drop basketball-size parachute flares, larger and brighter than the Army's mortar and artillery flares. Brady picked one out and started to circle it with his ship, dropping lower and lower into the fog, rain, and mist. The flare's brilliant light reflecting off the fog and rain wrapped the Dust Off ship in a ball of luminous haze. Brady dropped still lower, gazing out of his open side window, alert for the silhouette of crags and peaks. Suddenly the ship broke through the clouds. Brady recognized the signal lights of the unit below him, and settled his ship onto the side of the mountain. He picked up the casualties and took off. Now that he was under the clouds he could see better, and he managed to fly back to Chu Lai at low level. Back at the base the rain was so heavy he could hardly see to land. While the patients were being unloaded, and the ship readied for a second trip out to the mountains, the 54th's commander, Lt. Col. Robert D. McWilliam, went out to Brady's ship and through the left window and asked the copilot how it was going. The young lieutenant just shook his head and said he couldn't believe it. Knowing that the man was gung-ho, McWilliam thought he would not leave the ship until the mission was over. He asked him, "Would you like me to take over for you?" Instantly the man was out of the aircraft, and McWilliam took his place.

As he and Brady flew back to the mountains, the ground controller vectored them into the middle of the thunderstorm. Lightning flashed around them, but Brady flew on to the pickup site, where he again managed to get down through the clouds using the Air Force flares. But this time he could not find the 101st patrol before the flares burnt out. Flying around in the dark only a few hundred feet off the valley floor, he and McWilliam strained to see the signal light of the beleaguered unit. Just as they saw it, an enemy .50-caliber machine gun opened fire on them. Brady jerked his craft around to avoid the fire, and he and McWilliam lost the signal. Having lost the enemy fire as well, they circled for several minutes trying to find the signal again. Suddenly the .50-caliber opened up at them again, and Brady knew that the U.S. forces had to be near. He managed to stay in the area this time, and soon the signal light flashed again. The Dust Off ship landed and flew out more casualties.

Dust Off pilots often used Army artillery flares to light their pickup zone. But Major Brady had performed a far from standard night mission, using Air Force flares to descend through fog and rain in the mountains. In an article he wrote for *Army Aviation Digest,* Brady noted that such a mission did have its dangers, especially if the flares burned out before the ship had broken through the clouds. He wrote: "Nothing is more embarrassing than to find yourself in the clouds at 1,500 feet in 3,000-foot mountains and have the lights go out." The pilot's only recourse then was to climb as steeply as possible; if he tried to maintain position while waiting for another flare to come down, he ran the risk of drifting into the side of a mountain. Brady had demonstrated two qualities—imagination and courage—that helped many Dust Off pilots cope with the challenges of combat aeromedical evacuation.

Enemy Fire

Although pilot error and mechanical failure accounted for more aircraft and crew losses in Vietnam than enemy fire, the air ambulance pilots worried more about the latter danger than the othe more controllable ones. Once the buildup got under way in 1965, any air ambulance pilot who served a full, one-year tour could expect to have his aircraft hit by the enemy at least once. When hoist missions became a routine part of air ambulance work in late 1966, enemy fire became especially dangerous. Although the pilots devised ways of reducing the danger, such efforts barely kept pace with improvements in enemy weaponry and markmanship.

Before the buildup began the pilots had little more than homemade weapons to fear. In 1962 and 1963 the 57th Air Ambulance Detachment suffered less from enemy fire than the nonmedical helicopter units, partly because of the limited number of missions the unit flew in this period. The unit's five ambulance helicopters flew a total of only 2,800 hours those two years, and no pilot or crewman was wounded or killed in action. To get their minimum flight time and provide themselves some insurance against a lucky enemy hit, the pilots started flying two ships on each mission. But once the buildup got under way in late 1964 the unit went back to single ship missions, and most of the division and nondivisional air ambulance units that later joined them also followed this practice.

The return to single-ship missions demanded a few unorthodox procedures. International custom and the Geneva Conventions, which the United States considered itself bound to observe, dictated that an ambulance not carry arms or ammunition and not engage in combat. But in Vietnam the frequent enemy fire at air ambulances marked with red crosses made this policy unrealistic. Early in the war the crews started taking along .45-caliber pistols, M14 rifles, and sometimes M79 grenade launchers. The ground crews installed extra armor plating on the backs and sides of the pilots' seats. The hoist missions, introduced in the late fall of 1966, produced a high rate of aircraft losses and crewmember casualties. Although at this stage of the war gunship escorts for air ambulance missions were still hard to arrange, only the Air Ambulance Platoon of the 1st Cavalry responded to the new danger by putting machine guns on their aircraft. At first the unit simply suspended two M60's on straps from the roof over the cargo doors. Later they installed fixed mechanical mountings for the guns. A platoon aircraft also usually carried a gunner as a fifth crewmember to handle one of the M60's. Later in the war many of the air ambulance units, both divisional and nondivisional, tried to arrange gunship escorts, especially for hoist missions, to pickup zones that had been called in as insecure. Throughout the war, however, such escorts proved hard to obtain, because aeromedical evacuation was always a secondary mission for a gunship in a combat zone.

None of these defensive measures reduced the rate of air ambulance losses in the war; they only prevented it from approaching a prohibitive level. Most of the Viet Cong and North Vietnamese soldiers clearly considered the air ambulances just another target. A Viet Cong document captured in early 1964 describing U.S. helicopters read: "The type used to transport commanders or casualties looks like a ladle. Lead this type aircraft 1 times its length when in flight. It is good to fire at the engine section when it is hovering or landing." Fortunately Viet Cong weapons early in the war made a helicopter kill virtually impossible. Late in 1964, however, the North Vietnamese began to supply the Viet Cong with large amounts of sophisticated firearms: Chinese Communist copies of the Soviet AK47 assault rifle, the SKS semiautomatic carbine, and the RPD light machine gun. The introduction of these new enemy weapons in 1965–66 and of the hoist missions in late 1966 caused a dramatic increase in 1967 in the rate of enemy hits on air ambulances. Only in April 1972, however, when the United States was well along in turning the war over to the South Vietnamese, did the air ambulance have to contend with the Soviet SA–7 heat-seeking missile. This antiaircraft device was about five feet long, weighed thirty-three pounds, and had a range of almost six miles. A pilot had little warning of the missile's approach other than a quick glimpse of its white vapor trail just before it separated the tail boom from his aircraft. This weapon downed several air ambulances in the last year of U.S. participation in the war.

The missile also disrupted the most elaborate effort the Army made during the war to reduce the losses of air ambulances: a change of their color. The 1949 Geneva Conventions did not require that air ambulances be painted white, and for their first nine years in Vietnam the Army's air ambulances were the standard olive drab, medically marked only by red crosses on small white background squares. Early in the war many of the pilots thought that the crosses improved the enemy's aim at their ships, and the unit commanders had to resist pressure to remove the markings. Arguing that they would be unable to keep aircraft that looked like transports dedicated to a medical mission, the commanders prevailed, and the red crosses remained for the rest of the war.

By mid-1971, however, the high loss rate for air ambulances over the last six years produced much doubt about the olive drab color scheme. Believing that making the aircraft more distinctive might be the answer, the Army Medical Command in Vietnam secured approval in August to paint some of its aircraft white. The Command also was allowed to try to persuade the enemy that the white helicopters were for medical use only and should not be fired on. Thousands of posters were to be distributed and millions of leaflets dropped over enemy-held territory. The most elaborate leaflet read

Some new medical helicopters not only have Red Cross markings on all sides but they also are painted white instead of green. This is to help you recognize them better than before in order to give the wounded a better chance to get fast medical help. Like all other medical helicopters, these new white helicopters are not armed, do not carry ammunition, and their only mission is to save endangered lives without distinction as to civilians or soldiers, friend or foe.

• •

MEDICAL HELICOPTERS ARE USED FOR RESCUE MISSIONS AND THEY ARE NOT ENGAGED IN COMBAT. YOU SHOULD NOT FIRE AT THEM.

An enemy soldier still intent on bringing down any U.S. helicopter would now find the white helicopters excellent targets against a background of forests, hills, or mountains. All armaments now had to be removed from the ambulances, and gunship escorts could no longer furnish close support. Unless the information campaign were successful, the air ambulances would encounter more rather than less resistance. But the risk, while undeniable, seemed justifiable in view of combat loss statistics: from January 1970 through April 1971 the air ambulance combat loss rate was about 2.5 times as great as that for all Army helicopters. Something had to be done.

The test program for white helicopters, begun on 1 October 1971, soon produced encouraging preliminary results. In November the Army medical command received permission to paint all of its remaining fifty air ambulances white. However, the drawdown of U.S. forces was now in full swing. The test, which terminated the following April, had begun too late in the conflict and with too few helicopters to produce conclusive results. The white helicopters at least had not proven any more dangerous than those painted olive drab. On 28 April 1972 the MACV Surgeon recommended to the Surgeon General that white helicopters continue to be used for medical evacuation by the dwindling number of Army units in Vietnam.

But in the same month the enemy's introduction of the heat-seeking SA7 missile to South Vietnam put Army medical planners in a new quandary. To navigate properly, most air ambulance pilots could not fly to and from a pickup zone at altitudes low enough to enable the enemy on the ground to discern the white color and the red crosses. Except at the pickup zone, the white ambulances were as vulnerable as any other Army olive drab aircraft. Between 1 July 1972 and 8 January 1973 the enemy fired eight heat-seeking missiles at white air ambulances. The only protection against the SA7 was a new paint that reflected little of the engine's infrared radiation but dried to a dull charcoal green. In January 1973 USARV/MACV Support Command directed that all U.S. Army air ambulances in Vietnam be painted with the new protective paint. Research began on a white protective paint, but before any significant progress could be made the war ended.

A Turning Point

By early 1968 the basic techniques of aeromedical evacuation developed during the Vietnam War had been perfected. The helicopters, rescue equipment, and operating procedures were now ready for a full test of their utility. Their first trial came in February 1968 when the enemy launched a coordinated assault on allied bases and population centers throughout the country. With little warning the Dust Off system had to cope with thousands of casualties in all four Corps Zones. The enemy offensive resulted in more helicopter ambulances being shipped to South Vietnam, and by January 1969 the system was only one platoon short of its peak strength. That year Dust Off carried more patients than in any other year of the war. Although the fighting then began to wane for U.S. forces, the Dust Off system still had to face two more ordeals: large operations in Cambodia and Laos. The final years of Dust Off in Vietnam proved to be the most difficult, and they earned helicopter evacuation a lasting place in modern medical technology.

CHAPTER V

From Tet To Stand-Down

A reconsideration of the Vietnam War in 1968 by the American people and their government led to the withdrawal of U.S. combat forces from most of Southeast Asia by March 1973. After reports of a vast enemy offensive in South Vietnam in February 1968 reached the American public and the Johnson administration, support for the war, already less than firm, quickly waned. Although the coordinated enemy attacks heavily damaged several allied facilities and caused many casualties, the enemy itself suffered greatly in this futile attempt to topple the American-backed Republic of Vietnam. All in all, 1968 proved to be a near military disaster for the Viet Cong and their North Vietnamese allies. But once the United States began to withdraw from South Vietnam by the end of the year, events on the battlefield had less and less influence on the overall American military policy in that country. This last and most trying period of the American experience in Vietnam severely tested the courage and dedication of the U.S. Army's combat troops, including its Dust Off pilots and crews.

Tet — 1968

By the end of 1967 the enemy had staged large attacks on the border areas at Song Be, Loc Ninh, and Dak To. The enemy had done much the same in February 1954, just a month before the opening of the final campaign at Dien Bien Phu. Their strategem almost worked again. In early December 1967 Generals Westmoreland and Cao Van Vien, chief of the South Vietnamese Joint General Staff, discussed the coming Christmas, New Year, and Lunar New Year (Tet) ceasefires. In a show of confidence on 15 December, Westmoreland transferred the responsibility for defending Saigon to the ARVN forces and began to move large numbers of U.S. troops outside the Saigon area. But in early January the allies intercepted a message instructing the rebel troops to flood the Mekong Delta, attack Saigon, and launch a general offensive and uprising. On 10 January Westmoreland, after hearing the advice of Lt. Gen. Fred Weyand, the commander of II Field Force, Vietnam, began shifting combat units back from the border areas to Saigon. By 20 January U.S.

strength in Saigon had almost been restored to its previous high level. Westmoreland warned his superiors that the enemy might attack before or after the Tet holiday, which would last seven days starting 30 January, but he doubted that they would violate the traditional holiday truce itself.

On 20 January the enemy started their final diversion: a bombardment of the U.S. Marine Base at Khe Sanh in northern I Corps Zone. This siege continued some eleven weeks, well beyond the collapse of the Tet offensive, and demanded a large-scale rescue effort by U.S. forces in the north. On the morning of 30 January, the start of the Tet holiday, some Viet Cong units prematurely attacked seven cities. The main enemy attacks began the next day throughout the country and continued through 11 February. Although the allied command on 30 January cancelled all holiday leave for military personnel, few soldiers returned to their posts quickly enough to help stem the main attacks. The enemy failed to provoke a national uprising, and suffered heavy losses. But the Tet offensive damaged many allied, especially South Vietnamese, facilities and caused thousands of allied civilian and military casualties.

Enemy attacks on allied bases quickly drew Dust Off into the thick of the fighting. In the north the 43d Medical Group suffered damage to many of its dispersed aircraft. All medical units, both north and south, had been warned at least a few hours in advance to expect heavy casualties, but the offensive still almost swamped all allied hospitals and clinics. On 1 February the 43d Medical Group, with the 44th Brigade's approval, requested a C–141 for a special mission, evacuating as many U.S. casualties as possible from the 6th Convalescent Center, the 8th Field Hospital, and the 91st Evacuation Hospital, to make room for the continuing influx of wounded. CH–47 Chinook helicopters evacuated many patients between hospitals and casualty staging facilities.

On 1 February the 44th Medical Brigade's aviation officer told the various medical groups that all helicopter ambulance detachments were limited to twelve pilots, regardless of any other authorization. Both pilots and machines had become critically short. If any of the 43d's detachments should run into severe problems, it was to turn to the 55th Group and the 498th Medical Company. Later the 43d Group did have to call on the 55th Group for substitute aircraft. Only the somewhat sporadic nature of the fighting allowed the medical system to keep up with the inflow of patients.

At the start of the Tet offensive, the air ambulance detachments in the south were no better prepared for the onslaught of wounded than those in the north. The 44th Brigade began to keep constant watch on the status of the aircraft with each detachment so it could redistribute the flyable aircraft to the detachment in greatest need. But fighting soon inflicted a great deal of damage to the Dust Off aircraft throughout South Vietnam.

The problems of the 45th Medical Company and the 57th Detachment, both stationed at Long Binh outside Saigon, were typical. By midday on 1 February both units had notified the 67th Medical Group that they needed a hospital to receive ARVN patients, but the only one with any beds still open was at Vung Tau, sixty-five kilometers from Saigon on the coast. Since the 45th was down to seven flyable aircraft of its complement of twenty-five, the 44th Brigade gave it two aircraft from the 43d Medical Group. By the time the fighting subsided, twenty-two of the 45th's aircraft had been damaged. Some administrative delays were avoided during the fighting when the 67th and 68th Medical Groups allowed the 45th Company to coordinate directly with the 57th for such mutual support as they needed.

Tet swept through the Delta as it did elsewhere. The 82d Medical Detachment at Soc Trang had to support the U.S. 9th Infantry Division, three ARVN divisions, the 164th Aviation Group, and scattered Special Forces units. In February the pilots evacuated over 1,400 patients. The unit lost three aircraft the first night of the offensive. First up that night, Capt. Harvey Heuter, flew to Can Tho to pick up three casualties, then proceeded to Vinh Long for more, on his way to the 3d Surgical Hospital at Dong Tam. Vinh Long was wrapped in close-up fighting, even on the airstrip. After he left the strip with his first load, Heuter radioed his unit that from the air the friendly soldiers were indistinguishable from the enemy; he recommended the front of the dispensary as the safest place for the next helicopter to land for the rest of the casualties. While gunships orbited and fired when they could clearly see enemy on the ground, another 82d ship, piloted by Capt. Al Nichols, flew into Vinh Long and out again, taking fire both ways. The 82d often had to borrow aircraft, and sometimes it used pilots from other units to keep up with the missions.

Whereas most of the fighting in the Tet offensive lasted only a few days, the fighting in the ancient city of Hue, near the coast in northern I Corps Zone, raged for twenty-five days. The Army's 1st Cavalry Division had started moving north in January to conduct joint operations with the U.S. Marines and possibly to take part in a relief operation toward the Marine base at Khe Sanh. The Air Ambulance Platoon moved with them to the airstrip that served Hue and adjacent Phu Bai. After one night at Phu Bai the Air Ambulance Platoon pitched their tents in an area nearer Hue that they appropriately named "Tombstone"—their base was in a graveyard. The same area later became Camp Eagle when the 101st Airborne set up its division base there. After a few nights at Tombstone, and a few Viet Cong mortar attacks, the platoon moved north with the 1st Cavalry to a new base,

Camp Evans, a former Marine base along Route 1 toward Quang Tri. The platoon then dispersed its twelve aircraft among five locations.

On the morning of 31 January some seven thousand enemy soldiers, mostly North Vietnamese regulars, swarmed over Hue and seized all of the city except the Imperial Palace and the MACV compound across the Perfume River. Maj. Dorris C. Goodman, the platoon commander, and Capt. Lewis Jones pulled the first evacuation mission out of Hue. They low-leveled down the Perfume River into the city. At the pickup site, they found that the patients were not yet ready. After flying back to the River, they hovered between two gunships until called back in to complete the pickup. They then low-leveled out the way they had come in. Other Medevac ships followed them along the same route in the days of fighting that followed. As in the south, the air ambulances proved how necessary they were. Landing on tops of buildings and in city streets, using their hoists for inaccessible areas, the crews flew round the clock, not only to evacuate the wounded but also to move patients from overcrowded hospitals to other medical facilities. The Air Ambulance Platoon, the 571st Medical Detachment, and elements of the 498th Medical Company took part in Operation PEGASUS, a joint allied operation in early April to relieve the Khe Sanh combat base.

One of the most dramatic Dust Off missions in the north came shortly after a platoon of the 101st Airborne on the night of 3 April set up camp about five miles southeast of fire support base Bastogne on Highway 547 west of Hue. The mountains around them were dark, drenched with rain, and covered in fog. About 0100 the enemy probed the camp's perimeter with automatic weapons fire, then launched a ground attack. It was quickly beaten off, but two U.S. soldiers were critically wounded. The platoon leader called for Dust Off and specified that the mission required a hoist. The 101st Brigade Surgeon monitored the call and advised Dust Off to wait until daybreak to attempt the mission, since to fly that night with no visibility would court disaster. Lieutenants Michael M. Meyer and Benjamin M. Knisely cranked as soon as the mission request came through again at dawn. They set up a high orbit while waiting for the C-model gunships to fly out from Hue to cover them, but the gunships radioed they could not get out because of the fog. Meyer made a low pass over the area and, although the platoon leader did not mark his position with smoke, Meyer's crew made a fairly good identification by radio. The ground unit told Dust Off they had received a few rockets and considerable small arms fire, and they suggested he wait for guns to cover the mission. Meyer returned to Phu Bai to refuel and get his gun team.

At noon the Dust Off ship started out again to pull the two original casualties and three newly wounded soldiers, but this time with two UH–1C gunships alongside. Once in the area, the gunships made several passes in the vicinity of the platoon to draw fire, but they took none. Meyer shot his approach up the valley and came to a hover. The medical corpsman and crew chief had trouble seeing down through the trees. Finally the corpsman said he could see people on the ground and started the hoist cable on its way down.

Just then the gun team leader saw a trail of white smoke streaking toward the red cross on the fully opened cargo door, but before he could radio a warning a rocket struck and exploded. The aircraft, engulfed in flames, half flew, half bounced almost a quarter of a mile down the tree-covered hillside. The last thing Knisely remembered was the cargo door flying past his window. His helmeted head struck the door jamb and he passed out. The burning ship crashed down through the trees and came to rest on its left side. Meyer climbed out of the ship and started running, but stopped when he heard screaming, and returned. He kicked out the windshield, reached in, and unbuckled the unconscious Knisely who fell forward against the instrument panel. As he did so, a fuel cell in the belly of the ship exploded and blew Meyer away from it. He returned a second time, removed Knisely's helmet and pulled him from the ship. With his bare hands he patted out the burning jungle fatigues and then dragged his inert pilot a safe distance away. Before he could return to see if the crew were still alive, machine gun rounds started cooking off and the ship completely burned, an inferno of magnesium and synthetics. Later that afternoon Knisely regained consciousness, but neither of the pilots wanted to move very far. The ship was no more than a pile of ashes.

About 1700, hearing sounds of people approaching, Meyer and Knisely, both injured and unarmed, could do no more than crawl further under the bushes. From the voices, they immediately decided their visitors were not of English extraction. Just as the North Vietnamese troops arrived, an American rescue party also appeared and a skirmish broke out. For twenty minutes bullets whizzed and whined overhead and around the smoldering ashes of the Dust Off ship. The North Vietnamese finally broke contact and escaped down the hill.

The downed crew heard voices calling out in English. They were still afraid to answer but Meyer finally called out. The patrol was from the platoon—a lieutenant, a radioman, a medical corpsman, and several soldiers who had volunteered to work their way down the hill to the crash site and to rescue any survivors. They had not expected to run into the North Vietnamese patrol. It had taken them five hours to get to Meyer and Knisely. The corpsman checked them both over carefully: both of Meyer's hands were burned and one was broken, and Knisely had third-degree burns on one arm, lesser burns on his face, and a broken ankle. The trip back up the hill to the defensive perimeter was torturous for all concerned. Knisely, only intermittently conscious, could not walk and had to be carried or dragged.

The group made only a few hundred meters that first night.

While clambering up the hill the next morning, they heard shouting from overhead. They looked up a nearby tree and saw the medical corpsman, who had been thrown from the aircraft as it careened down the hillside. The party got him down and found that he had a broken hip and various bruises and contusions, but altogether he was a very lucky lad. The crewchief, Sp4c. James E. Richardson, had perished in the inferno of the crash.

Early that afternoon, the rescue party and the three Dust Off survivors rejoined the platoon where they learned that one of the gunshot victims had died. Because the enemy was still around in force, Dust Off could not get into the area without hazarding another loss. The downed crew told the ships overhead that it was not really urgent to get them out. They spent a second night on the ground.

Next day, when Lt. Col. Byron P. Howlett, Jr., the 498th's commander, heard of the crash, he and one of the platoon leaders jumped into an aircraft and flew the three hours from Qui Nhon to Phu Bai to hasten the extraction. Once there, Colonel Howlett declared that he was going to pull the mission no matter what. The next morning, he flew out and orbited the area with several gunship escorts to protect the attempt. One of the gunships dropped several blocks of plastic explosive so that the platoon below could blast out a landing zone. But the trees proved too dense to clear much more than a 30-by-30-foot area, far too small for a Huey to land in. By noon all the platoon and the crew were in the middle of the clearing. A Skyraider made several passes on the hill near the clearing, followed by Huey gunships. Then Dust Off, piloted by Howlett, flew in, hoisted out the three most serious casualties, all from the 101st, and evacuated them to the clearing station at Bastogne. A 571st ship flew in next, hoisted out several more wounded, and departed. On the third extraction, Colonel Howlett pulled Meyer and Knisely. The two ships had hoisted twenty-three wounded.

The Drawdown Begins

The war changed considerably after the enemy defeat during the Tet Offensive of 1968. By the end of the year many North Vietnamese units had withdrawn to Cambodia and Laos, leaving behind smaller units to harass the allied forces. The Military Assistance Command responded by adopting new tactics for its ground forces, using small units against precise objectives rather than large forces on area sweeps. These changes, however, did not immediately affect the well-established system of medical evacuation. By the end of the year air ambulance coverage was at its peak. Though the 50th Detachment was deactivated on 1 July, it soon reappeared as the twelve-helicopter

Air Ambulance Platoon of the 326th Medical Battalion, 101st Airborne Division (Airmobile), in northern I Corps Zone. The platoon quickly became known as Eagle Dust Off, the second air ambulance platoon in South Vietnam, joining the Medevac platoon of the 1st Cavalry.

In 1969 the war changed in several important ways. The diplomats in Paris conducting peace negotiations, which had begun after Tet, put procedural questions aside and began to concentrate on substantive issues. Ho Chi Minh died and was replaced by a collective leadership in North Vietnam. In the United States, the administration of President Richard M. Nixon, facing ever stronger domestic opposition to the war, announced the first of a series of withdrawals of U.S. troops from Vietnam. In March 1969, U.S. forces in Vietnam totaled 541,000, the peak level of American involvement. But in June, September, and December, President Nixon announced phased withdrawals of 110,000 U.S. personnel. The United States told the Republic of Vietnam that eventually it would have to defend itself without the aid of American ground combat forces.

The changes in the war produced changes in the Army's system of medical care. In the summer of 1969, the 44th Medical Brigade was removed from the 1st Logistical Command and assigned directly to U.S. Army, Vietnam. Eliminating that link in the chain of command greatly increased the brigade's influence. As combat and support units began to leave South Vietnam, U.S. troop locations and assignments changed rapidly, demanding equally rapid reassessments and readjustments of the medical support structure. Hospitals closed, reduced their holding capacity, or relocated. Coordination at the MACV level and between the various service components became vital.

In the summer of 1969, the 44th Medical Brigade deactivated the 55th Medical Group, which had never commanded aeromedical evacuation units, and thereby reduced its groups in Vietnam to three: the 67th in I Corps Zone, the 43d in II Corps Zone, and the 68th in III and IV Corps Zones. On 15 January 1970 the 44th Brigade further reduced its medical groups by deactivating the 43d at Nha Trang. The 67th Group at Da Nang then assumed control of I Corps Zone and the northern half of II Corps Zone; the 68th Group at Bien Hoa took the southern half of II Corps Zone along with III and IV Corps Zones. At that time the 44th Brigade exercised command and control over all U.S. Army medical resources in South Vietnam, except for those organic to combat units. The USARV Surgeon General's office existed as a separate staff element under USARV headquarters. Since this produced much duplication of function and effort, on 1 March 1970 the headquarters of the 44th Medical Brigade and the USARV Surgeon's office merged to form the U.S. Army Medical

Command, Vietnam (Provisional) (MEDCOM). The MEDCOM commander, Brig. Gen. David E. Thomas, also held the position of USARV Surgeon.

A Second Medal of Honor

Even as the drawdown got under way, in October 1969 Dust Off showed that its pilots could be heroes in times of withdrawal. CW3 Michael J. Novosel, a pilot of the 82d Medical Detachment, 45th Medical Company, 68th Medical Group, stationed at Binh Thuy in the Delta, seemed an unlikely hero. Forty-eight years old and a father of four, he was in his second tour of duty in Vietnam. In 1964 he had abandoned a lucrative pilot's job with Southern Airways and the rank of lieutenant colonel in the Air Force Reserve to serve as an Army pilot in Vietnam, where he joined the Dust Off team. Four times a day he applied medication to his eyes to treat the glaucoma whose onset had recently prevented him from returning to work as a civilian airline pilot. Only because the Army had granted him a waiver for his condition was he now back in Vietnam, again serving as a Dust Off pilot. Standing only five feet four inches, weighing less than 150 pounds, he lacked the physical characteristics of the stereotypical military hero. But he possessed qualities that were more important than physical prowess.

On the morning of 2 October 1969 the right flank of a three-company ARVN force came under intense fire as it moved into an enemy training ground right on the Cambodian border in the Delta province of Kien Tuong. During the next six hours U.S. Air Force tactical air support and Army gunships tried several times to enable the stranded soldiers to escape. Most of the uninjured soldiers managed to retreat some two thousand meters south, but others, finding their retreat blocked by high waters in swamps and rice paddies, could not get out. Several who had been wounded lay scattered about where they had been hit, near a group of bunkers and two forts used by the enemy in training exercises for simulated attacks on South Vietnamese installations.

In the midafternoon a U.S. Army command-and-control helicopter above the battleground radioed for a Dust Off ship. Operations control of the 82d Detachment relayed the request to Dust Off 88, whose aircraft commander, Mr. Novosel, and pilot, W01 Tyrone Chamberlain, had already flown seven hours of missions that day. The crew chief was Sp4c. Joseph Horvath and the medical corpsman was Sp4c. Herbert Heinold. Norosel immediately headed toward the border. Since the wounded ARVN soldiers did not show themselves on his first two hotly contested approaches to the area, Novosel circled at a safer range to signal the wounded to prepare for an evacuation.

Finally one soldier had the nerve to stand up in elephant grass and wave his shirt overhead. Novosel dropped his ship into the area again and skidded along the ground toward him. The crew scooped the soldier up and took off.

After that, by ones and twos, the ARVN soldiers waved to the circling helicopter that continued to draw enemy fire. Four soldiers stood up and Dust Off 88 picked them all up on one approach. Enemy machine guns killed at least one other soldier as he signaled. At 1730, Dust Off 88 dropped the first load of casualties off at the Special Forces camp at Moc Hoa, refueled, and headed back to the fray. While Chamberlain monitored the instruments and tried to spot the casualties, Horvath and Heinold hung out both sides of the aircraft on the skids, grabbing people when they could and pulling them inside the ship. Where the elephant grass was so tall that it prevented landing, Horvath and Heinold hung onto litter straps to reach far enough down to grab the men below.

During the second series of lifts, while Novosel hovered at a safe range, Air Force F-100's roared down on the enemy, dropping 500-pound bombs and firing 20-mm. cannon. But when Dust Off 88 went back in for the wounded, enemy fire was still extremely intense.

The second group of ARVN soldiers were seriously wounded. One had a hand blown apart; another had lost part of his intestines; another was shot in the nose and mouth. As soon as the ship left the area for Moc Hoa, Heinold began tending the more seriously injured, applying basic lifesaving first aid, to make sure the wounded were breathing and that the bleeding was momentarily stanched. During the fifteen minute flight back he also managed to start intravenous injections on those he thought were low on blood or going into shock.

Although the enemy fire knocked out the VHF radio and airspeed indicator early in the mission, Novosel continued to fly. At least six times enemy fire forced him out of the area. Each time he came back in from another direction, searching for gaps in the enemy's fixed field of fire from the fort and numerous bunkers. Between his three trips to the area Novosel used his craft to guide the withdrawal of stragglers around the swamps and rice paddies.

On the last of his trips, with dusk approaching, a pair of AH-1G Cobra gunships gave the helicopter some covering fire. At 1900, when nine casualties were already on board, Horvath told Novosel that a man close to a bunker was waving to them. Suspecting that something was awry, Novosel told his crew to stay low in the ship while he hovered backwards toward the man, putting as much of the airframe as possible between the bunker and his men. As soon as the soldier was close enough, Horvath grabbed his hand and started pulling him into the ship. Before he could get him in, an enemy soldier stood up in the grass about thirty feet in front of the ship. He opened fire with his

AK47, aiming directly at Novosel. Bullets passed on either side of him. One deflected off the sole of his shoe, and plexiglass fragments from the windshield hit his right hand. Shrapnel and plexiglass buried in his right calf and thigh. Both in pain and disgust, and to warn the copilot, Novosel shouted, "Aw hell, I'm hit." The aircraft momentarily went out of control and leaped sixty feet into the air. The ARVN soldier Horvath had been pulling aboard slipped off the ship, but Horvath kept his grip and pulled him back in. As he did so, he fell backwards on some of the men already there and cut his neck on their equipment. Chamberlain got on the aircraft controls with Novosel and they flew back to Moc Hoa. They shut down the engine, unloaded the wounded, and inspected their ship. Despite several hits to the rotor system and the cockpit, the aircraft could fly. The crew returned to Binh Thuy, ending their work after eleven hours in the air. They had evacuated twenty-nine wounded ARVN soldiers, only one of whom died. For this, Novosel was awarded the Medal of Honor.

VNAF Dust Off

In spite of the bravery of Army Dust Off pilots like Mr. Novosel, the Vietnamization of the war required that the South Vietnamese Army rapidly develop its own Dust Off system. The United States in May 1956 had taken responsibility for training and advising the South Vietnamese Air Force. The United States soon supplied the Vietnamese with H–19 helicopters, and later replaced them with H–34's. In August 1965 the Vietnamese Air Force received U.S.-made B–57 Canberra bombers, its first jet aircraft. In October of the same year it received its first UH–1B's. By the end of 1972, as a result of Vietnamization, it owned 500 new helicopters, organized in eighteen squadrons—"one of the largest, costliest, and most modern helicopter fleets in the world." By July 1972 U.S. flight schools in the continental United States had graduated 1,642 South Vietnamese helicopter pilots. No materiel or personnel shortages prevented the creation of an effective VNAF Dust Off system.

From the very first years of Dust Off in Vietnam, Army regulations specified that the primary responsibility for aeromedical evacuation of ARVN casualties lay with the South Vietnamese Air Force. ARVN officers were supposed to refer missions to the U.S. medical regulators only when their Air Force could not fly the mission. But in practice this regulation was often ignored. In November 1968 the USARV commanding general cabled all Army commands in the country: "Attempts to supplant VNAF with USARV resources or to allow requests for medevac of ARVN troops to go directly to USARV elements without first asking for VNAF precludes the RVN from developing effective aeromedical evacuation capabilities. Commanders are enjoined to prohibit such attempts."

Medical Command, Vietnam, responded to this directive by changing several elements of USARV Regulation 40-10, concerning aeromedical evacuation, to try to prevent Dust Off from accepting Vietnamese missions except when the case was urgent and the RVN Air Force fully committed elsewhere. The only civilians to be evacuated were those in the Civilian War Casualty Program. But the problem would not go away. A MEDCOM staff officer wrote to the Surgeon General's office: "It is definitely an uphill fight mainly because VNAF controls the aircraft and our USAF are their advisors. Our USAF has gone on record stating that dedicated aircraft for battlefield evacuation is ridiculous and a waste of assets. This policy has made it impossible to get our foot in the door thus far."

In February and March 1969 several U.S. commanders in Vietnam urged the creation of a Dust Off training program for VNAF pilots and medical corpsmen. One commander even suggested giving the RVN Air Force thirty-six new helicopters if they would promise to dedicate them exclusively to air ambulance missions. Over the next two years several attempts to work out a plan for attaching VNAF pilots and medical corpsmen to American Dust Off units failed because of disputes between the U.S. Army and U.S. Air Force over the concept of dedicated aircraft, because of the seemingly intractable nature of the language barrier, and because of the reluctance of the RVN Air Force to accept responsibility for its own Dust Off program.

Finally on 3 March 1971, after almost two years of talks and four months of preparation, the 57th and 82d Medical Detachments in IV Corps Zone started a Dust Off training program for VNAF helicopter pilots and crews. The Americans soon observed that the VNAF pilots learned faster than was expected. The two detachments arranged a rest area for the VNAF crews, allowed them to eat at U.S. Army mess halls, but flew them back to their base at Binh Thuy, near Can Tho, at the end of the day. On 21 March the first all-VNAF crew flew out of Binh Thuy on a Dust Off pickup. By September the program had trained some fifty VNAF pilots and crews in Dust Off procedures. Similar efforts in the other Corps Zones were also successful. Between late May and the end of October a similar program at Long Binh could graduate only nine of the twenty VNAF pilots who started. Three of those who graduated, however, started training other VNAF pilots; so by the end of November VNAF Dust Off crews were flying 70 percent of the patients in III Corps Zone. Similar programs in I and II Corps Zones ended in early 1972 with good results. By January 1972 all four programs had trained eighty-three VNAF pilots, twenty-one crew chiefs, and twenty-eight medical corpsmen, all of whom were considered fully qualified.

In addition to this training program, the MACV Surgeon's office saw that the number of VNAF Dust Off aircraft increased in step with

Vietnamization. From 1 November 1971 to 30 April 1972, as a part of the overall U.S. withdrawal, the U.S. Army gave the South Vietnamese armed forces 270 UH–1H utility helicopters, 101 O–1G light observation helicopters, and 16 CH–47 Chinook transport helicopters. The MACV Surgeon's office tried to ensure that about 6.5 percent of VNAF helicopters would be permanently dedicated medical evacuation ships. MACV planners fully realized that this minimal allocation would be inadequate to cover civilian casualties and nonurgent military casualties as well as urgent military casualties. But they considered it the best they could hope for.

During this period of rapidly dwindling resources, the U.S. Army Dust Off program experimented with a new form of organization—the medical evacuation battalion—that proved to be more successful than the medical evacuation company. Plans for such a unit originated in July 1969, just as the first stand-downs from Vietnamization began to take place in the 9th Division. On 1 August, the 54th Medical Detachment (Helicopter Ambulance) at Chu Lai created a similar unit by taking over the operational control of a dental service team, a preventive medical team, a veterinary detachment, and the 566th Medical Company (Ambulance). Although this new organization provided professional services other than medical transportation, it foreshadowed the medical evacuation battalion by combining surface and air evacuation assets.

In February 1970 the 44th Medical Brigade started to convert the 61st Medical Battalion at Cam Ranh Bay into just such a battalion. The brigade stripped the 61st of its responsibility for treating patients, then relocated it northward to Qui Nhon. When it became operational on 26 February 1970, the 61st started to control all nondivisional ambulances in the northern half of South Vietnam. The mission of the battalion was considerably broader than that of a detachment or company; it had to provide ground as well as air transport, and move not only patients but also medical personnel, supplies, and equipment.

To accomplish this mission, the battalion had six helicopter ambulance detachments, two ground ambulance detachments, one bus ambulance detachment, and one air ambulance company—a total of sixty-one UH–1H helicopters, eighty-seven 3/4-ton ambulances, and three bus ambulances. To improve the command structure of the battalion, its commander formed smaller air ambulance "detachment groups." A MEDCOM aviation officer explained the rationale behind the action:

We are paying some high penalties because of the lack of experienced aviators. We just do not have enough second-tour types to provide a commander for each unit. Our average for both commissioned and warrant second tours is far below the USARV average. In an effort to compensate fo this lack of experience "Detachment Groups" have been formed, where two or more detachments are located in close proximity, with the senior aviator assigned controlling and coordinating activities. We hope this will give us better control and take maximum advantage of the experience we do have.

The 283d air ambulance detachment was put under the 498th Medical Company (Air Ambulance), the 236th and 237th air ambulance detachments under the 571st air ambulance detachment, and the 68th air ambulance detachment under the 54th air ambulance detachment.

The 61st Medical Evacuation Battalion proved successful. Aircraft availability rates increased 20 percent and the battalion's units passed their command inspections with flying colors. Plans were made for a second battalion. On 1 May 1970 the 58th Medical Battalion became the 58th Medical Evacuation Battalion, with its headquarters at Long Binh. Its mission was to provide coverage for southern II Corps Zone, and III and IV Corps Zones. The battalion had fifty-five UH–1H helicopters to support this area.

For a year the two evacuation battalions performed their tasks very well. But by the spring of 1971 the declining personnel ceilings in Vietnam had made the battalions an unaffordable luxury. Medical Command, Vietnam, prepared to deactivate the battalions and transfer many of their functions to the staff of the 67th and 68th Medical Groups. On 10 June both battalions totally disbanded.

Cambodia

From the early 1960s the North Vietnamese Army had brought supplies and troops into South Vietnam along the Ho Chi Minh Trail running south through the Laotian panhandle and eastern Cambodia, and along the trails running northeast from the Cambodian coast on the Gulf of Thailand. In 1967 the United States began covert operations, code-named SALEM HOUSE, against these enemy supply routes. Although limited in size and scope—each incursion team had a maximum of twelve allied soldiers, including three American soldiers, and a maximum penetration of twenty kilometers into Cambodia—some 1,400 SALEM HOUSE missions took place from 1967 through 1970.

In early 1970 the U.S. military leaders in Vietnam saw the need for larger strikes against the supply routes. Insurgents in Cambodia were stepping up their campaign against the new anti-Communist Cambodian government of Lt. Gen. Lon Nol, and Phnom Penh, the Cambodian capital, was soon isolated. On 1 April the Viet Cong and North Vietnamese forces began to clear a corridor ten to fifteen miles wide along the border all the way from the Gulf of Thailand to the

Fish Hook region north-northwest of Saigon, threatening III and IV Corps Zones in South Vietnam.

Responding to these threats, the allied forces decided to openly assist the new Cambodian government. In mid-April ARVN forces conducted a limited cross-border raid near the Parrot's Beak region, south of the Fish Hook region. At the same time U.S. and ARVN staffs started planning for a joint operation against several enemy sanctuaries in Cambodia, especially in the Fish Hook region, and on 28 April President Nixon approved the final plan. From early May to the end of June elements of several large U.S. combat units in South Vietnam—the 1st Infantry Division, the 1st Cavalry Division, and the 11th Armored Cavalry Regiment—took part in these joint strikes at suspected Viet Cong bases over the border. USAF B-52 tactical bomb strikes and large-scale U.S. helilifts and helicopter gunship strikes prepared the way for the ground forces.

Dust Off and Medevac helicopters supported both South Vietnamese and American soldiers in this operation. During May the 1st Cavalry's Air Ambulance Platoon supporting the attack flew 1,042 missions (307 in Cambodia) and evacuated 1,600 patients (946 from Cambodia). The dense jungle and forests along the border resulted in eighty hoist missions for 182 patients. Although constituting only 7.6 percent of the total missions for May, hoist missions accounted for 53 percent of the ships hit by enemy fire that month. In May four ships were destroyed and eleven damaged. Ten crewmen were wounded and one killed. In June deeper penetrations into Cambodia increased flying time for the pilots and crews, even while the number of missions declined as the fighting tapered off. The crews flew 682 missions (199 in Cambodia) and evacuated 1,056 patients (397 from Cambodia). They also extracted 185 patients in ninety-one hoist missions. The 45th Medical Company and the 159th Medical Detachment helped the Air Ambulance Platoon by backhauling many patients to hospitals around Saigon. Because the Viet Cong had been warned of the foray and had fled the area, casualties were far below the April estimates. What had loomed as a severe test for the Dust Off system proved to be largely routine work, except for the dangerous hoist missions over triple-canopy jungle and forest.

A Medevac in Peril

One of these hoist missions during the Cambodian operation demonstrated that the air ambulance pilots had no monopoly on heroism among the U.S. Army medical personnel in Vietnam. On the morning of 24 May 1970 a helicopter of the Air Ambulance Platoon was ferrying S. Sgt. Louis R. Rocco, the medical adviser of a MACV advisory team stationed at Katum. Since December 1969

Sergeant Rocco had served as liaison to the 1st ARVN Airborne Division's medical battalion. He had trained ARVN personnel on mission requests, use of the hoist, the forest penetrator, and the semi-rigid litter, and he also had presented classes on basic first aid. Whenever his duties allowed him the time, Rocco rode the medical helicopters on live missions to help the medical corpsmen and to practice some "hands on" medicine himself.

At 1100 on 24 May, Medevac 2 with Sergeant Rocco on board flew toward its base at Katum, in northern Tay Ninh province along the Cambodian border. A request for a pickup came in through the radio of a command-and-control helicopter flying overhead. The call was on behalf of eight urgent patients of the 1st ARVN Airborne Division. Two of the division's companies, the 61st and 63d, were on a sweep operation five miles inside the Cambodian border. The day before, the two companies had made contact with a North Vietnamese force that broke off and withdrew. The commander of the 61st Company had the small task force dig in for the night. The enemy attacked at dawn on the twenty-fourth but was repulsed by the defenders. In pursuing the North Vietnamese the ARVN soldiers took eight casualties. The U.S. advisers to the 61st and 63d Companies radioed their evacuation request through Maj. Jesse W. Myers, Jr., senior battalion adviser, who was overhead in a command-and-control helicopter.

The pilot of Medevac 2, 1st Lt. Stephen F. Modica, radioed that he would take the mission as soon as he dropped off a load of supplies. At Katum, the crew threw the beer and sodas onto the pad, grabbed an extra chest protector for Rocco, and took off again. Regulations of the 1st Cavalry required gunship cover for evacuation missions if a unit had been in contact with the enemy within the past twenty-four hours. Usually C Battery, 2d Battalion, 20th Aerial Rocket Artillery— the "Blue Max"— provided this cover by orbiting a team of two AH–1G Cobras, one high and one at treetop level. Medevac 2 had already learned from the U.S. adviser with the ARVN companies that the last contact had been to the north two hours earlier. Soon the Blue Max gun team arrived on station; Modica briefed them on the situation and said he would shoot his approach from the south. When the helicopter dropped to the landing zone, North Vietnamese hidden in the trees and along the ridge line opened fire with small arms and automatic weapons. The lower gunbird opened fire at the muzzle flashes in the trees. On its second pass it used its grenade launcher; the enemy redirected some of its fire and the gunship took its first hit. On its next run it again took enemy fire.

Just before the Medevac landed, two enemy rounds hit Modica in he chest protector and one passed through his left knee and lodged against the femur. As soon as the aircraft bumped down, the copilot turned to kid Modica that he ought to practice his landings. When he saw Modica's wounds, he took the controls and pulled the ship out of the landing zone. The aircraft rose fifty feet into the air before the engine stalled and the aircraft crashed back to the ground. Major Myers later described what he saw from above in his command-and-control ship: "The [Medevac] ship seemed to land, then shot up in the air, and then fell to the ground rolling over on its side, thrashing around like a wounded insect....Smoke was pouring out of the ship by this time...." The two gunships made low firing passes to give the Medevac crew a chance to get out, if any still lived. One Cobra gunship came to a high hover over the burning Medevac, spinning and firing at the North Vietnamese. The gunship took twenty-nine hits before its ammunition ran out, forcing it to depart. The pilot transmitted a Mayday for the downed Medevac, giving its location and identification, and then called Medevac Operations to repeat the information.

All the Medevac crew were stunned at first and unable to move. Finally Rocco dragged himself out and crawled away. He had a fractured wrist and hip and a severely bruised back. As soon as he realized that the crew was still inside, he went back. He pulled Modica through the shattered windshield and carried him across twenty meters of exposed terrain to the ARVN perimeter. One by one he brought the unconscious crew out. All were in bad shape. Modica had his serious leg wound. The copilot, 1st Lt. Leroy G. Cauberreaux, had a broken collar bone and fractured ribs. Sp5c. Terry Burdette, the medical corpsman, had a broken shoulder and a broken leg. The gunner, Sp4c. Gary Taylor, who sat in the right door, was crushed and burned when the ship crashed and rolled, and Rocco severely burned his hands trying to find him. The nearby ARVN soldiers could not help because the enemy was shooting at anyone who moved. The two bullets that hit Cauberreaux in the chest protector as Rocco carried him toward the ARVN perimeter did no further damage. Rocco had saved his three comrades from certain death.

At Quan Loi, the Air Ambulance Platoon's base, Capt. Henry O. Tuell III, aircraft commander of Medevac 1, yelled to his pilot, 1st Lt. Howard Elliot, that Modica had been shot down. Elliot was in the shower; he grabbed a towel and ran to get his clothes, scattering soapy lather as he went. By the time he had thrown his clothes on, Tuell had already cranked the aircraft; off they flew, Elliot lacing boots and fastening zippers. Although several other aircraft were in the area, Medevac 1 was the first evacuation ship on the scene. Medevac 2 was still burning, throwing off blankets of black smoke. Medevac 1 made its approach straight in and the enemy tried for another score. On each side of Medevac 1 two Cobras fired flechettes, machine guns, grenades, and rockets; but enemy rounds still hit the ship. One came through the left door and hit the armored seat just below Tuell's hand

Shrapnel and shattered porcelain from the seat peppered his hand and wrist. Elliot took the controls and nursed the ship back to Quan Loi where a doctor cleaned, stitched, and dressed Tuell's injuries.

Two hours later, after several air and artillery strikes around the perimeter, the pilot of Medevac 12, Lt. John Read, had his gunship escort lay down a heavy rocket preparation as he tried a highspeed, low-level approach to Medevac 2. The North Vietnamese, still safely bunkered behind 1½ feet of concrete, blasted Medevac 12 out of the area before it could land. Bullets punctured the fuel cells and disabled the engine. With his tachometer falling, Lt. Read managed to land his ship safely in a nearby clearing, where the crew was immediately picked up.

Back at the crash site Modica remained conscious despite loss of much blood, and talked to the aircraft orbiting helplessly overhead. The American adviser with the ARVN forces, S. Sgt. Louis Clason, told him that the ARVN soldiers had not been resupplied in two days and were running out of everything, including water. Modica told him, "Hey, listen. We have one case of beer in the tail boom of the aircraft. You run out there—at least that's something to drink." Clason told him, "Lieutenant, you don't even know what your aircraft looks like. It is burned completely to the ground." About 1800, Modica radioed the nearby aircraft that the ARVN defenders might not be able to hold on through the night. After an hour of continuous friendly shelling around the allied perimeter, Medevac 21, piloted by CWO Raymond Zepp and covered by gunships, made the third attempt to reach the downed aircraft. The Cobra fired a 360° pattern with rockets and miniguns, but enemy fire still riddled the Medevac, knocking out its radios and starting an electrical fire. Like Medevac 12, Medevac 21 landed in a field 500 meters to the west; its crew was quickly pulled out. Nightfall prevented any further rescue attempts.

During the long hours of darkness, the enemy launched three assaults on the small perimeter. Flares overhead illuminated the area and allowed the Americans to call in artillery and gunships to break up the ground attacks. By nightfall Rocco's injuries had immobilized him. After pulling his crew from the burning ship, he had treated their injuries and the ARVN casualties he could get to. Soon his injured hip and hand stiffened, making any effort to move excruciatingly painful. Finally he passed out. Modica's leg swelled to twice its normal size and the pain immobilized him too. Cauberreaux moved about and lit cigarettes for the men, but with his crushed right side he could do little else. Since they had no morphine or other painkiller, they had to suffer.

At Quan Loi, planning for an all-out rescue attempt continued well into the night. The plan called for two Medevacs to go in and evacuate Modica's crew and any South Vietnamese possible. A third would hover nearby to extricate the crews if trouble developed and to evacuate any remaining ARVN casualties. Since all their Medevacs were shot up, destroyed, or committed elsewhere, the 1st Cavalry had to borrow three nondivisional Dust Off helicopters. At 0930 next morning ARVN and American howitzer batteries started laying a barrage of smoke rounds in the area to create a screen for the upcoming rescue. Just before the operation began, four Cobras fired more smoke rounds. At 1145 the flight of three Medevacs with three cobras on each side started into the area. The first ship in loaded Modica and his crew and flew out. The second extracted several ARVN wounded and also safely left the area. An enemy rocket hit the third ship as it took off with two remaining ARVN casualties, but the crew brought the ship down without further injuries and was quickly rescued. The next day nine pilots and crewmen involved in this rescue received Silver Stars. Sergeant Rocco won a Medal of Honor for his part in saving Modica and most of his crew.

Laos

By October 1970 allied intelligence clearly showed two very disturbing facts. After recovering from the setback inflicted by the allied attack in Cambodia, the enemy was making plans to strangle Phnom Penh, depose the Lon Nol government, and reopen their southern supply routes by retaking the port of Kompong Som on the Gulf of Thailand. Also, the North Vietnamese Army was improving its road nets in Laos, building up supplies, and sending reinforcements, all apparently in preparation for large-scale offensives in I Corps Zone. Starting in early January 1971 the U.S. XXIV Corps and the South Vietnamese Joint General Staff began planning for a preventive strike on the enemy bases and lines of communication between the northwest border of I Corps Zone and the Laotian city of Muang Xepon. In keeping with President Nixon's Vietnamization program, the South Vietnamese Army was to supply the ground combat forces while the United States supplied air and artillery support. U.S. forces were forbidden to set foot on Laotian soil.

Laos turned into Dust Off's greatest test in the Vietnam war. The complexity and offensive character of the operation presented the allies a new problem: the helicopter transport and evacuation of large forces in rapidly changing tactical situations. From 8 February through 9 April 1971 U.S. aircraft, including Air Force B-52's and some 650 Army helicopters, transported ARVN troops into Laos, gave them covering fire, and evacuated their wounded and dead. The U.S. units involved were reinforced contingents from the 101st Airborne Division (Airmobile), 5th Infantry Division (Mechanized), and

23d ("American") Infantry Division. All operated under the command of Headquarters, XXIV Corps. The offensive accomplished one objective: it delayed the enemy at least several months. But it showed that even with U.S. support the ARVN forces lacked the leadership to prevent heavy losses — approximately 50 percent casualties.

The ARVN part of this joint, four-phased operation was called LAM SON 719; the U.S. part, DEWEY CANYON II. Between 30 January and 7 February the allies were to clear western Quang Tri Province and the east-west Route 9 as far west as the Laotian border, establishing forward U.S. bases at the abandoned Khe Sanh combat base and fire support base Vandegrift. In Phase II between 8 February and 6 March the South Vietnamese would cross the border into Laos, establish fire support bases, and press on to Muang Xepon. During the next three days, or Phase III, the South Vietnamese would locate and destroy enemy caches and installations in and around Muang Xepon. In Phase IV all forces would gradually withdraw from Laos either along Route 9 or along a more southern route.

All of this information was so tightly held for security reasons that medical planners were unaware of the impending operation until the last few days of January. Finally the XXIV Corps Surgeon, the senior medical adviser in I Corps Zone, and the commander of the ARVN 71st Medical Group received a partial briefing on the objectives and plan of execution. They set to work immediately, realizing that plans for medical support had to be hastily drawn up. Fortunately, both the ARVN and U.S. medical units had stockpiled considerable reserves of supplies in anticipation of a 1971 Tet offensive. Because of the paucity of information, casualty estimates had to be extremely rough. In fact, because of the minimal resistance expected from the supposedly rearguard enemy troops in the area, first predictions were for low casualties.

After the first briefings, the 67th Medical Group immediately began to give South Vietnamese units additional training in the use of U.S. medical evacuation. The ARVN interpreters assigned to work with the Dust Off crews were given as much training as the week's busy schedule permitted. After the 1st Brigade, 5th Infantry Division, completed its two-pronged drive west to Khe Sanh, it dug in at that base with two 101st Airborne Eagle Dust Off helicopters standing by. Khe Sanh served as the forwardmost site of medical support for the eleven U.S. battalions working between there and the border. The Dust Off helicopters also stood ready to assist the forty-two South Vietnamese maneuver battalions assigned to the operation. Dust Off helicopters backhauled U.S. casualties to the 18th Surgical Hospital at Quang Tri once they were able to travel. Two other Dust Off aircraft stationed at the 18th were to cover the land north to the Demilitarized Zone and west to the base named Rock Pile on Route 9. All four of these ships were committed to area support. On 5 February the 67th Medical Group put a liaison officer at the 18th Surgical to respond better to the needs of the U.S. forces.

Meanwhile the ARVN medical service set up its hospital eight kilometers south of Khe Sanh at Bach Son. The South Vietnamese set up tents and excavated bunkers. The facilities included two operating rooms, an X-ray room, and fifty underground beds. The main Vietnamese hospital for LAM SON 719 was near the coast, at Dong Ha, at the intersection of Routes 1 and 9.

The Laotian operation presented the problem of suddenly coordinating aeromedical evacuation units whose work so far had usually been at scattered sites and, especially in the detachments, under only tenuous control by superior organizations. Because of the dangers of the missions and the direct involvement of most of the resources of two air ambulance detachments—the 237th and the 571st—Col. Richard E. Bentley, commander of the 61st Medical Battalion and aviation staff officer of the 67th Medical Group, ordered that either the commander or operations officer of the 571st be physically present at the Khe Sanh operations bunker to help regulate both the 237th and 571st. This order stood until the difficulty of controlling both fixed and rotary-wing aircraft and coordinating them with artillery strikes, bombing, and ground maneuvers finally forced the XXIV Corps to request the 67th Medical Group for operational control of the two detachments. The 67th consented. The XXIV Corps assigned operational control of the detachments to the 326th Medical Battalion of the 101st Airborne, which then controlled the operations of all evacuation helicopters at Khe Sanh and Quang Tri. Two other MEDCOM Dust Off units, the 236th Detachment and the 498th Medical Company, also furnished general support for northern I Corps and helped backhaul patients from the 18th Surgical Hospital at Quang Tri and the 85th Evacuation Hospital at Phu Bai to the 95th Evacuation Hospital at Da Nang.

When Phase II of the operation began, two MEDCOM Dust Offs joined the Medevacs and Eagle Dust Offs camped at Khe Sanh to support the invasion. Two of the four ships were put under the operational control of the 101st Combat Aviation Group, primarily to cover combat assaults and pull downed crews from Laos. The U.S. medical staff quickly set up a few standard procedures for the incursion. Since no U.S. advisers would accompany the ARVN ground troops into Laos, all medical evacuation missions across the border had to have an ARVN interpreter on the aircraft. Once the heavy enemy antiaircraft defenses in Laos became apparent, the staff decided that gunships would have to cover the air ambulances once they crossed the border. Finally, all evacuation requests would have to pass through a tactical operations center, preferably that of the ARVN I Corps, rather than go directly to the aircraft commanders.

During the first three weeks of the operation, the air ambulance crews complained vociferously. The larger concept of the operation had not been made clear to them, and the lack of gunship cover, the poor communications, and the false information on area security and casualties suggested to them that the operation was a mess. The further the South Vietnamese penetrated into Laos, the more intense became the antiaircraft fire and the indirect fire on the landing zones. As Phase II drew to a close, however, some of the operating procedures smoothed out. Dust Off representatives now sat in the divisional tactical operations centers; ground commanders overcame much of their reluctance to talk with helicopters; and gunship cover became routinely available. Coordination of divisional and nondivisional air ambulances improved markedly once the evacuation requests were funneled to a single Dust Off operations center at Khe Sanh.

Efficiency suffered most of all from the bad weather. The area east of the mountains was still in the winter monsoon season. At the same time, the weather at Khe Sanh and to the west would often be flyable. Since it was on a high plateau, Khe Sanh itself often required instrument flight while the nearby areas were under visual flight rules. Often an aircraft took off from Khe Sanh in the late afternoon, flew a pickup from Laos, and then had to fly all the way back to Quang Tri to land because of poor visibility and low ceilings at Khe Sanh. On twenty-four of forty-four days of the Laos operation, low ceilings and reduced visibility delayed flight schedules. On some days there were no flights at all because of the weather.

Efficiency also suffered from the poor arrangements for backhauls. During Phase I of the operation, patients at Khe Sanh were placed on fixed-wing resupply ships for medically unattended flights south to Da Nang or Tan Son Nhut. But this practice was not sanctioned and ceased early. On 12 February at the request of the Surgeon of the U.S. XXIV Corps, the 101st Combat Aviation Group began furnishing two CH-47's each day to backhaul routine cases from the ARVN hospital at Bach Son. But this was inadequate; Dust Off aircraft at Khe Sanh still had to backhaul emergency cases to Dong Ha. As casualties mounted, the backhauls impaired Khe Sanh's ability to respond rapidly to requests for field evacuation. The medical system had control of too few aircraft to discharge all of its responsibilities.

Poor coordination of gunship support also became a key obstacle to air ambulance missions. On 24 February, mission response time rose to seven hours because of delayed gunship protection. Finally, after several complaints by the air ambulance crews, the 101st Airborne and the XXIV Corps agreed to dedicate some gunships to air ambulance coverage. When an air ambulance launched from Khe Sanh, the 101st Combat Aviation Group had gunships primed to go with it;

two teams were on standby during the day and one at night. The 101st Group also had a fire team positioned at Dong Ha for Dust Off protection. But gunship support for all the missions into Laos was still impossible, since there were not enough gunships available to satisfy all the high priority combat and medical missions. The problem continued until 25 February, when the XXIV Corps gave Dust Off the highest priority for gunship support regardless of the tactical situation or other requests. Even so, the enemy antiaircraft fire was so intense and the flight routes so restricted by weather and geography that many Dust Off crews resumed the old practice of flying all missions in pairs, to allow one crew to immediately recover its downed teammate.

North Vietnamese intelligence had given the enemy ample time to deploy an extensive, well-integrated, and highly mobile air defense system throughout the Xe Pon area of Laos. Many enemy antiaircraft weapons were radar-controlled, and Dust Off pilots monitoring their VHF radios came to recognize the "wheep wheep" of the radar sweeps and take evasive action. But the North Vietnamese had spread some 750 medium caliber antiaircraft machine guns along Route 9 and the valley of the Xe Pon River leading west to Muang Xepon. The North Vietnamese relocated most of their antiaircraft weapons daily, making their detection and destruction a difficult task.

The North Vietnamese also placed mortar, artillery, and rocket fire on every potential landing zone. Each zone was assigned a heavily armed team of ten to twelve men. Every airmobile operation, including what normally were single ship Dust Off missions, had to be worked out and coordinated, with fire support, armed escort, and a recovery plan. As soon as a mission request came in, a command-and-control ship, gunships, and the air ambulance would crank and launch. This medical evacuation package would rendezvous near the Laotian border and fly across. En route to the pickup, the command ship helped with navigation and steered the group around the antiaircraft sites. As it neared the destination, the air ambulance would thread its way through a corridor of friendly artillery, tactical air support, and gunships. While the ambulance was on final approach, on the ground, and departing, the gunships would circle overhead, giving nearly continuous protective fire. After the pickup, the group flew a different corridor back to Khe Sanh.

Papa Whiskey

One Dust Off mission during the Laos operation illustrated both its chaotic finale and the bravery of a Dust Off crewman. On 18 February a North Vietnamese regiment assaulted fire support base Ranger North, nine kilometers inside Laos. About 1130 the South Vietnamese 39th Ranger Battalion holding the base asked the Dust

Off operations center at Khe Sanh to evacuate its many seriously wounded. A Dust Off aircraft, with a crew from both the 237th and 571st Detachments, took off and headed west. On their first attempt to land they took such heavy fire that the commander, CW2 Joseph G. Brown, aborted his approach. A second time around he tried a high speed descent and made it in. Just before the ship touched down the enemy opened fire again and continued firing while the crew loaded the wounded Rangers. Uninjured Rangers trying to escape the base also poured into the ship, and Brown had trouble lifting it off. Just as he cleared the ground, a mortar round exploded in front of the cockpit, shattering the console and wounding him. The ship crashed. Rangers scattered from the wreck and the Dust Off crew dragged Brown to a ditch for temporary shelter. Leaving him with his pilot, CW2 Darrel O. Monteith, the crew chief and two medical corpsmen started running toward a bunker. A mortar round exploded and blew one corpsman, Sp4c. James C. Costello, to the ground. His chest protector had saved his life, and he stood up, shaken but uninjured. The same explosion blew shrapnel into the back and left shoulder of the crew chief, Sp4c. Dennis M. Fujii. A second mortar round wounded the other corpsman, Sp4c. Paul A. Simcoe. The three men staggered into the bunker.

Shortly before 1400 an Eagle Dust Off ship tried to rescue them, but automatic weapons fire drove it off, wounding its pilot. At 1500 another Eagle Dust Off ship landed under heavy gunship cover. The wounded Dust Off crew, except for Fujii, raced to the Eagle ship. A mortar barrage falling around it kept him pinned in his bunker, where he waved off his rescuers. To escape the enemy fire the Eagle pilot had to take off, leaving Fujii as the sole American on the fire base, which was now surrounded by two North Vietnamese regiments. Another Dust Off ship soon arrived to pick up Fujii, but enemy fire forced it to return to Khe Sanh.

At 1640 Fujii found a working PRC–25 radio and started broadcasting, using the call sign "Papa Whiskey." He told the pilots high overhead that he wanted no more attempts to rescue him because the base was too hot. Using what medical knowledge he had picked up, he began tending to the wounded Rangers who surrounded him.

That night one of the North Vietnamese regiments, supported by heavy artillery, started to attack the small base. For the next seventeen hours Papa Whiskey was the nerve center of the allied outpost, using his radio to call in and adjust the fire of U.S. Air Force AC–130 flare ships, AC–119 and AC–130 gunships, and jet fighters. Working with the Air Force's forward air controllers, he coordinated the six flareships and seven gunships that were supporting Ranger North. Twice during the night the enemy breached the perimeter, and only then did Fujii stop transmitting to pick up an M16 and join the fight.

With the Ranger commander's permission, Fujii brought the friendly fire to within twenty meters of the base's perimeter, often leaving the safety of his bunker to get a closer look at the incoming friendly rounds. He worked all night and into the next morning, bringing in more than twenty coordinated gunship assaults.

The next afternoon an all-out rescue attempt began. A fleet of twenty-one helicopters descended on the base, the gunships firing on every possible enemy position. With Fujii also calling in artillery strikes, the allies ringed the camp with continuous fire. Even so, hostile fire was so intense that the commander of the rescue fleet, Lt. Col. William Peachey, prepared to send down a single ship rather than risk a formation. Fujii asked that as many of the 150 ARVN casualties as possible be evacuated before him, but Peachey ordered him to jump on the first ship that landed. Maj. James Lloyd and Capt. David Nelson left the formation, descended into the valley, then flew up a slope to the fire base, hugging the trees, and dropped in unharmed. Fujii scrambled on board with fourteen Rangers. Having recovered from their surprise, the enemy opened fire on the ship as it lifted off. Raked with bullets, it caught fire and the cockpit filled with smoke. The pilots headed toward Ranger South, fire base of the 21st Ranger Battalion about four kilometers southwest. They landed and everyone jumped from the burning ship as its M60 rounds started to cook off in the flames. Miraculously, no one was injured. Ranger South itself soon came under heavy enemy attack, but Fujii's work was over. Finally, at 1600 on 22 February, 100 hours after he was wounded, he was admitted to the 85th Evacuation Hospital at Phu Bai. He had helped save 122 Rangers. He was quickly awarded a Silver Star, which was later upgraded to a Distinguished Service Cross.

Fujii's mission was only part of an operation that had turned into an embarrassing scramble to safety. According to the after action report of the 61st Medical Battalion: "During the last phases of Operation Lam Son 719 enemy activity further intensified. Landing zones were dangerously insecure. Air Ambulances landing to pick up wounded were swarmed with fit and able soldiers seeking a way out of their increasingly precarious position. Medical evacuation pilots reported complete lack of discipline during the last days of the operation coupled with extremely hazardous conditions." Evacuation ships, and indeed any aircraft landing near the South Vietnamese units, were rushed by throngs of able-bodied soldiers trying to escape. One Eagle Dust Off ship, a UH–1H with a normal load of eleven passengers, landed for a pickup and had to take off almost immediately because of small arms fire and mortar rounds in the landing zone. After the pilot set his ship down in Khe Sanh, his crew counted thirty-two ARVN soldiers on board, all without weapons or equipment, on–

ly one of whom was wounded. To prevent ARVN soldiers from hitching a ride back on the sides of the aircraft, some crews resorted to coating the skids with grease.

By early April the Dust Off and Medevac ships had saved hundreds of lives. In the two-month operation they flew some 1,400 missions, evacuating 4,200 patients. Six crewmen were killed and fourteen wounded. Ten air ambulances were destroyed, about one out of every ten aircraft lost in the operation. On 8 April, once the incursion was over, XXIV Corps gave up its operational control of the MEDCOM air ambulances. Dust Off pilots had seen their last major operation of the war.

Stand-Down and Ship Out

The phased withdrawal of American forces from Vietnam, begun in the summer of 1968, continued until, on 11 August 1972, the last American ground combat unit stood down at Da Nang. The American venture in this small, remote Asian country had come full circle. More than seven years earlier, on 8 March 1965, the first U.S. ground combat forces had landed on these same beaches. In December 1961 the first U.S. military units, two helicopter companies, had arrived in Saigon to aid the South Vietnamese government. It had been the longest war in United States history, and almost half of it had been devoted to the withdrawal.

The drawdown of medical support paralleled that of combat forces, but lasted a little longer because of continuing medical needs of noncombat U.S. forces in Vietnam. In the early months of 1972 MEDCOM air ambulances decreased from forty-eight to thirty, leaving five detachments: the 57th, 159th, 237th, 247th, and 571st. In June 1972 the Air Ambulance Platoon of the 1st Cavalry stood down, leaving all air ambulance missions to the few remaining nondivisional Dust Off units. In February 1973 three of the last four Dust Off detachments—the 237th, 247th, and 571st—stood down. In February the 57th Detachment, the first to arrive in Vietnam and whose early commander, Maj. Charles Kelly, had created the Dust Off mystique, prepared to become the last to leave, closing down its operations at Tan Son Nhut. On 11 March it flew the last Dust Off mission in Vietnam, for an appendicitis case.

After they turned in their aircraft on 14 March, the few remaining members of the 57th had little to occupy their time. Some simply took pleasure in building their sun tans. A few tried to readjust their daily rhythms to Stateside time; they reset their clocks and began to live at their home hours, though this meant getting up in the dark and sleeping part of the day. Every now and then they had to check on their departure date, but no one demanded any work of them. On 28

March they received orders to move to Camp Alpha, the personnel staging facility at Tan Son Nhut, where they were restricted to the compound pending their flight out. Finally, at 0100 on the twenty-ninth, they boarded buses for a ride to their C–141 transport. The drivers halted the buses some fifty feet from the floodlighted jet, and kept the bus doors closed while a double file of people formed between the bus and the boarding stairs. The two lines were composed of Americans, South Vietnamese, North Vietnamese, and Viet Cong, all members of the Four Power Joint Military Commission that was supervising the implementation of the peace treaty.

The bus door opened, and one at a time the departing personnel of the 57th marched through this double file. They had been part of the last U.S. Army operational personnel in South Vietnam. The same day the Military Assistance Command, Vietnam, lowered its flag and ceased to function for the first time since 1962. The ground war in Vietnam was completely in the hands of the Republic of Vietnam for the first time in twenty-seven years. During a long, cruel, and ultimately losing struggle, Dust Off personnel had comported themselves with courage and honor, proving that a band of brave and dedicated pilots and crewmen could make this new mode of medical evacuation work extremely well, even against well-prepared enemy ground fire.

Epilogue

The Vietnam War had its precedents in American military history. At the turn of this century the U.S. Army in the Philippines, only a few years after the end of its trials during the Indian Wars of the American frontier, again fought an enemy that often used guerrilla tactics. In 1898 many American soldiers serving in Cuba suffered the torments of tropical disease. World War II in the Pacific, although conventional in nature, once more subjected American soldiers to the hardships of warfare in the tropics. But advances in weapons and military transport made the Vietnam War a virtually new experience for the American armed forces.

This was especially true for the Army Medical Department. Its experiences with patient evacuation in the Korean War had only foreshadowed the problems it would confront in South Vietnam. Helicopter ambulances in Korea had rarely needed to fly over enemy-held areas, and the terrain of Korea, although rugged, lacked the thick jungles and forests that obstructed the air ambulances in Vietnam. While Army hospitals in Korea had been highly mobile, moving often with the troops, the frontless war in Vietnam resulted in a fixed location for almost all hospitals. French armed forces had used the helicopter for medical evacuation in their unsuccessful struggle in Indochina, but since they had used aircraft that were soon obsolete, their experiences could offer little guidance to the Americans who arrived in Vietnam in 1962.

Statistics

Records produced by the various U.S. Army air ambulance units in Vietnam show that the Medical Department's new aeromedical evacuation system performed beyond all expectation. Although figures are lacking for some phases of the system's work, enough reports have survived to permit an assessment of what it accomplished. It is possible both to describe the number and types of patients transported and to compare the risks of air ambulance missions with those of other helicopter missions in the Vietnam War.

Air ambulances transported most of the Army's sick, injured, and wounded who required rapid movement to a medical facility, and also many Vietnamese civilian and military casualties. From May 1962 through March 1973 the ambulances moved between 850,000 and

900,000 allied military personnel and Vietnamese civilians. The Vietnamese, both civilian and military, constituted about one half of the total; U.S. military personnel, about 45 percent; and other non-Vietnamese allied military, about 5 percent. These proportions varied, however, over the course of the war. Before 1965 about 90 percent of the patients were Vietnamese. Then the U.S. buildup began in 1965, and the figure dropped to only 21 percent for 1966. As the United States started to turn over more of the fighting to the South Vietnamese, the number rose until it reached 62 percent in 1970. Unfortunately, exact percentages of wounded, injured, and sick among the air ambulance patients are lacking. Although only about 15 percent of the cases treated by all Army medical personnel in the war were wounded in action, it seems that the percentage of wounded among the air ambulance patients was much higher, between 30 and 35 percent, since the ambulances gave first priority to patients in immediate danger of loss of life or limb, a condition most closely associated with combat wounds. Up to 120,000 of the U.S. Army wounded in action admitted to some medical facility—90 percent of the total—were probably carried on the ambulances. This is about one third of the some 390,000 Army patients that the air ambulances carried to a medical facility.

The widespread use of the air ambulances clearly seems to have reduced the percentage of deaths from wounds that could have been expected if only ground transportation were used. In World War II the percentage of deaths among those Army soldiers admitted to a medical facility was 4.5; in Korea, 2.5. In Vietnam it was 2.6, despite a road network as bad as that in Korea, despite thick jungle and forest that made off-the-road evacuation much more difficult than in Korea, and despite the large numbers of hopeless patients whom the air ambulances brought to medical facilities just before they died. Another statistic—deaths as a percentage of hits—shows more clearly the improvement in medical care: in World War II it was 29.3 percent; in Korea, 26.3 percent; and in Vietnam, only 19 percent. Helicopter evacuation was only one aspect of the Army's medical care in Vietnam, but without that link between the battlefield and the superbly staffed and equipped hospitals, it seems likely that the death rate would have surpassed perhaps even that in World War II.

Measured both by the patients moved and the number of missions flown, the air ambulances were busiest in 1969, when by the end of the year 140 were stationed around the country. Over the course of the war the divisional air ambulances of the 1st Cavalry and 101st Airborne constituted only 15 percent of the total. Because of the high maintenance demands of the UH–1, only about 75 percent of the ambulances were flyable at any given moment, although replacement aircraft could sometimes be borrowed from helicopter maintenance companies. Of the aviators required by the Army tables of organization and equipment, an average of 90 percent was available for duty. Although at times the air ambulances were filled to capacity and even overcrowded, a single mission on the average moved only two patients. In the peak years of U.S. involvement, from 1965 to 1969, a single mission averaged, round trip, about fifty minutes. In the same period the ambulance units used the hoist only once every sixty missions. The helicopters averaged about two missions per workday in 1965, increasing to four missions in 1969.

Statistics also confirm the impression that the air ambulance pilots and crewmen stood a high chance of being injured, wounded, or killed in their one-year tour. About 1,400 Army commissioned and warrant officers served as air ambulance pilots in the war. Theirs was one of the most dangerous types of aviation in that ten-year struggle. About forty aviators (both commanders and pilots) were killed by hostile fire or crashes induced by hostile fire. Another 180 were wounded or injured as a result of hostile fire. Furthermore, forty-eight were killed and about two hundred injured as a result of nonhostile crashes, many at night and in bad weather on evacuation missions. Therefore, slightly more than a third of the aviators became casualties in their work, and the crew chiefs and medical corpsmen who accompanied them suffered similarly. The danger of their work was further borne out by the high rate of air ambulance loss to hostile fire: 3.3 times that of all other forms of helicopter missions in the Vietnam War. Even compared to the loss rate for nonmedical helicopters on combat missions it was 1.5 times as high. Warrant officer aviators, who occasionally arrived in South Vietnam without medical training or an assignment to a unit, were sometimes warned that air ambulance work was a good way to get killed.

One air ambulance operation, the hoist mission, added greatly to these dangers. Although hoist missions were rarely flown, one out of every ten enemy hits on the air ambulances occurred on such occasions. Standard missions averaged an enemy hit only once every 311 trips, but hoist missions averaged an enemy hit once every 44 trips, making them seven times as dangerous as the standard mission. That some 8,000 aeromedical hoist missions were flown during the war further testifies to the bravery of the air ambulance pilots and crewmen.

Doctrine and Lessons Learned

When the first Army air ambulances arrived in Vietnam in April 962, none of the existing Army guidelines for aeromedical evacuation fitted their needs. Only in August 1963 did the 57th Medical Detachment receive a mission statement, in the form of USARV Regulation 59-1 (12 August 1963). It contained a list of patient priorities, based on nationality and civilian-military status. It prohibited the use of the air ambulances for nonmedical administrative and logistical purposes, and it outlined the steps to be taken by ground commanders in making a request for an air ambulance. As the war progressed, the regulation was updated periodically to cover various emerging problems. By the end of the war it was twice as long as the August 1963 version, and it elaborated on several problems that had been ignored or treated only briefly in the original—hoist operations, evacuation of the dead, pickup zones reported as insecure, and misclassification of patients. A new category of patient had been designated: tactical urgent, meaning that the evacuation was urgent not because of the patient's wound but because of immediate enemy danger to the patient's comrades. The old categories of urgent, priority, and routine were now defined at length. An appendix and a diagram outlined the requesting unit's responsibilities in preparing a pickup zone. Little was left to the ground commander's imagination.

In spite of this amplification for the benefit of the ground commander, much was still left to the interpretation of the air ambulance commanders and pilots. Controversies over the use of the air ambulances that had surfaced early in the war were at its end untreated and unresolved by any Army regulation or field manual.

One of these problems concerned the best type of organization for air ambulance units. In an article in the August 1957 issue of *Medical Journal of the United States Armed Forces,* Col. Thomas N. Page and Lt. Col. Spurgeon H. Neel, Jr., had outlined current Army doctrine on aeromedical evacuation. One of their precepts read: "The company-type organization for the aeromedical function is superior to the current cellular detachment concept." But the first two aeromedical evacuation units that deployed to Vietnam were detachments that depended on nearby aviation units for their mess and other logistical needs, and for part of their maintenance. Although two TOE air ambulance companies, the 45th and 498th, were eventually deployed most of the air ambulances in the war worked in cellular detachments.

After the war several former aviation consultants to the Surgeon General stated that the company structure had provided administrative and logistical advantages that outweighed its disadvantages. Most former detachment commanders and some of the former company commanders, however, emphasized the weakness of the company structure. Because of the dispersed nature of the fighting in Vietnam, the platoons of the companies often were field-sited far from their company headquarters, creating a communication problem and also reducing the effectiveness of the company's organic maintenance facilities that were located at the home base. The detachments however, had their own limited maintenance facilities, and the pla toons organic to an airmobile division could readily draw on its resources. For about one year toward the end of the war an experiment with two medical evacuation battalions had produced encouraging results, but the experiment apparently was too limited to firmly establish the battalion as the ideal medical evacuation unit. No formal statement from the Surgeon General had resolved the issue by the end of the war: a policy of flexibility seems to have evolved by default, allowing the use of whatever type of organization best fitted the geographic region and phase of the war.

In 1957 Page and Neel had also written: "The consensus is that there is no real requirement for a separate communications net for the control of aeromedical evacuation." But the air ambulance units in Vietnam quickly found that tactical command networks were often too busy to permit their use by medical personnel. In September 1966 the commander of the 3d Surgical Hospital wrote: "Casualty control and medical regulating of patient load would be well served by a separate radio net exclusive to the medical service. Accurate knowledge of incoming loads of patients would allow proper notification of hospital personnel and preparation of critical supplies in advance. Multiple switchboards and untrustworthy landlines now prevent the dissemination of information which might aid in the optimal care of patients." Shortly thereafter the USARV regulation on aeromedical evacuation was amended to assign the air ambulance units two frequencies, one for use in I and II Corps Zones and one for III and IV Corps Zones.

In another area, Page and Neel had outlined a point of Army medical doctrine that remained, despite some complaints by combat commanders, inviolate throughout the war: "Within the Army, the Army Medical Service has the basic technical responsibility for all medical evacuation, whether by surface or aerial means . . . . The Army Medical Service requires sufficient organic aviation of the proper type to enable it to accomplish its continuing mission of rapid evacuation of the severely wounded directly to appropriate medical treatment facilities." The Medical Service received its helicopters in the buildup from 1965 through 1969, and most of the aviators who served as air ambulance commanders, whether commissioned or warrant officers, had received medical training comparable to that given a battalion surgeon's assistant. Only in the first years of the war were the detachments under the operational control of nonmedical aviation units. Medical control of air evacuation did not preclude having nonmedical aviation units evacuate large numbers of patients with only routine wounds, injuries, and illnesses. Page and Neel had written: "The Army Medical Service does not require sufficient organic aviation for the entire Army aeromedical evacuation mission .... The movement of nonemergency patients by air can be accomplished economically by making use of utility and cargo aircraft in conjunction with normal logistic missions, provided there is adequate medical control over the movement of patients." The twenty-four air ambulances of the 1st Cavalry and 101st Airborne Division also remained outside the jurisdiction of the Army medical command in Vietnam. Even so, all officer and most warrant officer ambulance pilots of the divisions had to pass the Medical Service Corps training program for ambulance pilots; and when the division pilots flew patients directly to a hospital, they were required to radio a 44th Medical Brigade regulating officer for approval of their destination.

While some combat commanders objected to medical control over evacuation of their casualties, others resented their inability to subordinate the Dust Off air ambulances to a mission of close and direct support for their particular unit. Although there was usually a considerable difference in rank between the aircraft commander of a Dust Off ship and the irritated ground commander, there apparently were few instances of the commander succeeding in obtaining direct support without first routing his request through prescribed channels. Throughout the war most Army commanders knew that casualties properly classified as urgent would almost always benefit from evacuation in an air ambulance.

One subject not touched upon by Page and Neel proved to be a source of lasting trouble in Vietnam. While the three basic patient classifications—routine, priority, and urgent—survived in the Army regulation until the end of the war, no agreement could be reached on the proper definition of these terms. Most of the controversy dealt with the category "priority," which as originally worded applied to a patient who required prompt medical care not available locally and who should be evacuated within twenty-four hours. In practice, the aeromedical units found that this definition often resulted in overclassification of priority patients as urgent patients, who were expected to be moved immediately. Most ground commanders simply would not take the responsibility of saying that any of their wounded could wait up to twenty-four hours for medical treatment. When the air ambulance units proposed shortening the time limit on priority patients, some staff officers noted that in practice the ambulances were picking up priority patients as soon as possible and that almost no priority patient ever had to wait twenty-four hours for evacuation. So USARV headquarters changed the regulation to read: "Priority: Patients requiring prompt medical care not locally available. The precedence will be used when it is anticipated that the patient must be evacuated within four hours or else his condition will deteriorate to the degree that he will become an urgent case." Even after this amendment, the regulation drew criticism from Maj. Patrick Brady, who argued that there should be only two categories: urgent and nonurgent. He thought that all missions should be flown as urgent, resources permitting, and that the requestor should be allowed to set his own time limit on nonurgent patients.

This controversy arose partly from the tension between those aviators who, preserving the Kelly tradition, paid scant attention to the security of the landing zone, the weather, or the time of day in deciding whether to accept a mission, and those units and aviators who adopted a cautious approach. The USARV regulation and the published operating procedures of some of the units favored the more cautious approach, calling for gunship escorts on all hoist missions, discouraging night missions except for urgent patients, and prohibiting flight into an insecure pickup zone. Night, bad weather, and reports of recent enemy fire in a pickup zone would keep the cautious pilots from even lifting off on a mission. But none of these would prevent the bolder pilots from making an immediate liftoff, even for a routine patient. Little short of enemy fire would keep the braver pilots, once they were above the landing zone on an urgent or priority mission, from going in. On an urgent mission, a few pilots like Major Kelly, Major Brady, and Mr. Novosel, would even fly into the teeth of enemy bullets to get to wounded. The bolder pilots also adhered closely to the section of the Geneva convention that required all air ambulances to carry no weapons. Although almost all the pilots took along sidearms, many declined the use of gunship escorts or externally mounted M60 machine guns.

The tension between these two approaches to air ambulance work could hardly have been resolved by any command edict, and no attempt was made to do so. The USARV regulation left the ultimate decision on whether to reject or abort a mission entirely in the hands of the individual aircraft commander who received the request. On Brady's first tour in Vietnam, one of his comrades told him that if he kept on taking so many risks he would either be killed or win the Medal of Honor. Consciously preserving the Kelly tradition, and drawing on his vast store of skill and luck, Brady survived and indeed won the nation's highest military award. Most of the pilots, while not quite measuring up to the Kelly tradition, acted bravely and honorably enough to win widespread respect and gratitude from those who served in Vietnam.

A Historical Perspective

What did the Dust Off experience mean to the history of medical evacuation? The concepts developed in Maj. Jonathan Letterman in 1862 — medically controlled ambulances and an orderly chain of evacuation that takes each patient no farther to the rear than necessary — are still sound. There will always be a hierarchy of medical facilities in wartime: the more specialized the care, the more likely it will be infrequently used, and centralized at a point well to the rear of a battlefront, often completely outside the war zone. Modern technology has made it possible to improve enormously the quality and range of care provided at hospitals in or near a war zone, especially in the area of lifesaving equipment and techniques. But the more complicated demands of restorative and recuperative care will probably long remain a duty of medical facilities in the communications zone and the zone of the interior. Helicopter evacuation and modern medical technology have only modified, not destroyed, the value of Letterman's system, particularly in medical care close to the scene of battle.

Because helicopter ambulances usually kept a combat unit within a half hour's flight time from an allied base in Vietnam, it was no longer necessary to set up the traditional hierarchy of medical facilities — a Letterman chain of evacuation. Battalion aid stations and division clearing stations found many of their old duties assumed by immobile and often distant surgical, field, and evacuation hospitals, where most patients, except those in remote areas such as the Central Highlands, were flown directly from the site of wounding. The speed of the helicopter ambulances combined with a proficient medical regulating system after 1966 allow the larger hospitals to specialize in certain types of wounds. Despite these advantages, the simplification of the Letterman chain of evacuation also had its dangers. At times, as during the battle around Dak To in 1967, the nearest hospitals able to take casualties might be too far away to permit direct flights from the battlefield. In times of large-scale casualties, such as the Tet offensive of 1968, central medical facilities unsupported by the triage and surgical services of lower echelon medical facilities, even if there were adequate warning, could find themselves overwhelmed. Sometimes, as during the strike into Laos in 1971, faulty casualty estimates could result in a local shortage of medical helicopters. Furthermore, the less seriously wounded patients of an air ambulance, especially those not requiring major surgery, could often find themselves evacuated farther to the rear than necessary.

Whether the modification of the Letterman system that occurred in Vietnam saves money — by specializing wound care, fixing the location of most surgically equipped hospitals, and reducing the care furnished at the division clearing stations and some of the smaller surgical hospitals — is debatable, given the attendant need to upgrade the larger hospitals in the combat zone and expand the expensive helicopter evacuation system. A more important question is whether the modification improves medical care and saves lives. The Dust Off story suggests that it did help reduce the Army's mortality rate in Vietnam. But it is doubtful whether that experience, in an undeveloped country and in a war against an enemy with few effective antiaircraft weapons, would prove wholly applicable in a large-scale conventional conflict in a more developed theater. In such a conflict there might be a role for truly mobile surgical hospitals, which were not used in Vietnam. Working close to the front, such hospitals would be within range of both ground and air ambulances. The ideas of Jonathan Letterman would still merit the closest attention.

Bibliographical Note

For sources the authors relied mainly on records produced by air ambulance units in Vietnam. Those records that have not yet been transferred to the National Archives, Record Group 112, Office of the Surgeon General, are stored in the Washington National Records Center, Suitland, Maryland.

Captain Dorland interviewed fifty-three people who took part in Dust Off operations in Vietnam. Dr. Nanney, in the final stages of preparing the manuscript, especially Chapter 4, interviewed the aviation consultant to the Surgeon General, Lt. Col. Thomas C. Scofield. Tapes of these interviews are available at the Center of Military History.

Most of the authors' sources were official records, but several articles, books, and official studies proved useful.

Articles

Binder, James L. "Dean of the Dust-Offers." *Army* 21 (August 1971): 16–21.

Brady, Patrick H. "Dust Off Operations." *Army Logistician* 5 (July-August 1973): 18–23.

_____. "Instruments and Flares." *United States Army Aviation Digest* 15 (January 1969): 12–13.

_____. "Solo Missions." *United States Army Aviation Digest* 12 (July 1966): 2–6.

Breese, J.E. "Rotors over the Jungle: No. 848 Naval Air Squadron in Malaya." *Flight,* 12 March 1954, pp. 291–92.

Clark, D.M. "Helicopter in Air Evacuation." *The Air Surgeon's Bulletin.*

Cooling, B. Franklin. "A History of U.S. Army Aviation." *Aerospace Historian* 21 (June 1974): 102–09.

Decker, Bill. "Medic." *Army Digest* 22 (July 1967): 27–29.

Eiseman, B. "The Next War: A Prescription." *United States Naval Institute Proceedings* 101 (January 1975): 33–40.

Farrell, Robert. "Special Report from Algeria, Part I: French Meet Guerrillas with Helicopters." *Aviation Week,* 17 September 1956, pp. 28–31.

_____. "Special Report from Algeria, Part II: Algerian Terrain Challenges Helicopters." *Aviation Week,* 24 September 1956, pp. 88–92.

Goodrich, Isaac. "Emergency Medical Evacuation in an Infantry Battalion in South Vietnam." *Military Medicine* 132 (October 1967): 796–98.

Haldeman, Steve. "Jungle Medevac." *Army Digest* 24 (August 1969): 44–45.

Harvey, E. Bruce. "Casualty Evacuation by Helicopter in Malaya." *British Medical Journal,* 1 September 1951, pp. 542–44.

Hasskarl, Robert A., Jr. "Early Military Use of Rotary Wing Aircraft." *Airpower Historian* 12 (July 1965): 75–77.

Hessman, James D. "U.S. Combat Deaths Drop 90 Percent as Vietnamization Takes Hold." *Armed Forces Journal* 109 (April 1972): 42–44.

Lam, David M. "From Balloon to Black Hawk." A four-part series. *United States Army Aviation Digest* 27 (June–September 1981).

Lawrence, G.P. "The Use of Autogiros in the Evacuation of Wounded." *The Military Surgeon,* December 1933, pp. 314–21.

"Missile! Missile! Missile!" *United States Army Aviation Digest* 21 (April 1975): 30.

Modica, Stephen F. "Medevac Meadow." *United States Army Aviation Digest* 21 (June 1975): 4–5.

_____. Letter to the Editor. *United States Army Aviation Digest* 21 (June 1975): 22–23.

Monnier, R., and G. Wernert. "Etat actuel de évacuations sanitaires par helicoptéres — Indochine." *Société de Médecine Militaire,* no. 4 (April 1956), pp. 116–23.

Neel, Spurgeon H. "Aeromedical Evacuation." *Army* 6 (April 1956): 30–33.

_____. and Roland H. Shamburek. "The Army Aviation Story: Part IX, Medical Evacuation." *United States Army Aviation Digest* 9 (February 1963): 33–41.

_____. "Dustoff: When I Have Your Wounded." *United States Army Aviation Digest* 20 (May 1974): 6–9.

_____. "Helicopter Evacuation in Korea." *United States Armed Forces Medical Journal* 6 (May 1955): 691–702.

_____. "Medical Considerations in Helicopter Evacuation." *United States Armed Forces Medical Journal* 5 (February 1954): 220-27.

Page, Thomas N., and Spurgeon H. Neel, Jr., "Army Aeromedical Evacuation." *United States Armed Forces Medical Journal* 8 (August 1957): 1195-1200.

Riley, David. "French Helicopter Operations in Algeria." *Marine Corps Gazette,* February 1958, pp. 21–26.

"Safety for Combat Readiness." *United States Army Aviation Digest* 15 (August 1969): 37–44.

Salvagniac, Surgeon General. "Les Evacuations Sanitaires Aeriennes." *Revue Historique De L'Armée,* no. 1 (1972): 230–53.

Scoles, Peter S. "Forward Medical Service of the Future." *Military Review* 41 (April 1961): 64–70.

Scotti, Michael J. "Out of the Valley of Death." *United States Army Aviation Digest* 16 (May 1970): 12–14.

Smith, Allen D. "Air Evacuation—Medical Obligation and Military Necessity." *The United States Air Force Air University Quarterly Review* 6 (Summer 1953): 98-111.

————. "Medical Air Evacuation in Korea and Its Influence on the Future." *The Military Surgeon* 110 (May 1952): 323–32.

Smith, William H. "Honor Times 29." *United States Army Aviation Digest* 20 (January 1974): 3–5.

"Treetop Whirlybird Nest." *Army* 15 (November 1965): 20–22.

"Up and Out." *United States Army Aviation Digest* 9 (September 1963): 13–16.

Wiegman, Curtis M. "To Save a Life." *United States Army Aviation Digest* 18 (August 1972): 56–59.

Williams, Charles. "Operations of the 1st Helicopter Ambulance Company." *American Helicopter* 32 (November 1953): 8.

Williams, Robert C. "Survivor Wishes to Meet Helicopter—Object: Survival." *United States Army Aviation Digest* 14 (May 1968): 55–59.

Books and Studies

Battelle Columbus Laboratories. *Journal of Defense Research: Series B (Tactical Warfare).* Vol. 7B, No. 3 (Fall 1975): *Tactical Warfare Analysis of Vietnam Data.* Especially Chapter XI: "United States Casualties Analyzed."

Bonds, Ray, ed. *The Vietnam War: The Illustrated History of the Conflict in Southeast Asia.* New York: Crown, 1979.

Collins, James L., Jr., Brig. Gen. *The Development and Training of the South Vietnamese Army, 1950–1972.* Department of the Army: Vietnam Studies. Washington, D.C.: Government Printing Office, 1975.

Department of Defense. "Report on Selected Air and Ground Operations in Cambodia and Laos." 10 September 1973. Army War College Library. Carlisle Barracks, Pa.

Kahin, George M., and John W. Lewis. *The United States in Vietnam.* New York: Delta, 1967.

Link, Mae Mills, and Hubert A. Coleman. *Medical Support of the Army Air Forces in World War II.* Office of the Surgeon General, United States Air Force. Washington, D.C.: Government Printing Office, 1955. Especially Chapter V: "Air Evacuation Missions," pp. 352–412.

Littauer, Raphael, and Norman Uphoff, eds. *The Air War in Indochina.* Air War Study Group, Cornell University. Revised edition. Boston: Beacon, 1972.

Neel, Spurgeon, Maj. Gen. *Medical Support of the U.S. Army in Vietnam, 1965–1970.* Department of the Army: Vietnam Studies. Washington, D.C., Government Printing Office, 1973.

Politella, Dario. *Operation Grasshopper: The Story of Army Aviation in Korea from Aggression to Armistice.* Wichita, Kansas: Robert Longto, 1958.

Stewart, Miller J. *Moving the Wounded: Litters, Cacolets, and Ambulance Wagons, U.S. Army, 1776–1876.* Ft. Collins, Co.: Old Army Press, 1979.

Tierney, Richard, and Fred Montgomery. *The Army Aviation Story.* Northport, Alabama: Colonial Press, 1963. Especially Chapter VI: "Medical Evacuation."

Tolson, John J., Lt. Gen. *Airmobility, 1961–1971.* Department of the Army: Vietnam Studies. Washington, D.C.: Government Printing Office, 1973.

Weinert, Richard P. *A History of Army Aviation, 1950–1962. Phase I: 1950–1954.* Fort Monroe, Virginia: U.S. Continental Army Command Historical Office, 1971.

Westmoreland, William C., General. *A Soldier Reports.* Garden City, N.Y.: Doubleday, 1976.

Index

☆ U.S. GOVERNMENT PRINTING OFFICE: 2008 346–747

ISBN 978-0-16-075478-4

9 780160 754784

90000

PIN: 083017